EXPERT GUIDE TO

ALLERGY AND
IMMUNOLOGY

To Amanda, Philip, Elena, & Alec

    May your days (and nights) be

sneeze & wheeze free.

          Grandpa

          4-12-99

For a catalogue of publications available from ACP–ASIM, contact:

Customer Service Center
American College of Physicians–American Society of Internal Medicine
190 N. Independence Mall West
Philadelphia, PA 19106-1572
215-351-2600
800-523-1546, ext. 2600

Visit our Web site at www. acponline.org

EXPERT GUIDE TO

ALLERGY AND IMMUNOLOGY

edited by RAYMOND G. SLAVIN, MD, FACP
and ROBERT E. REISMAN, MD, MACP

Foreword by Jerome P. Kassirer, MD, MACP

American College of Physicians
Philadelphia, Pennsylvania

Acquisitions Editor: Mary K. Ruff
Manager, Book Publishing: David Myers
Administrator, Book Publishing: Diane McCabe
Production Supervisor: Allan S. Kleinberg
Production Editor: Scott Thomas Hurd
Cover and Interior Design: Patrick Whelan

Printed in the United States of America
Composition by Fulcrum Data Services, Inc.
Printing/binding by Versa Press

American College of Physicians (ACP) became an imprint of the American College of Physicians–American Society of Internal Medicine in July 1998.

Library of Congress Cataloging-in-Publication Data

Expert guide to allergy and immunology / edited by
    Raymond G. Slavin and Robert E. Reisman.
        p.   cm. – (Expert guide series)
    Includes bibliographical references and index.
    ISBN 0-943126-73-8 (alk. paper)
    1. Allergy. 2. Immunologic diseases. I. Slavin,
Raymond G. II. Reisman, Robert E. III. Series.
    [DNLM: 1. Hypersensitivity. 2. Immunologic
Diseases.   WD 300E965 1999]
RC584.E97–dc21
616.6'1061–dc21
DNLM/DLC
for Library of Congress   98-28031
                                                                        CIP

The authors and publisher have exerted every effort to ensure that drug selection and dosage set forth in this manual are in accord with current recommendations and practice at the time of publication. In view of ongoing research, occasional changes in government regulations, and the constant flow of information relating to drug therapy and drug reactions, the reader is urged to check the package insert for each drug for any change in indications and dosage and for added warnings and precautions. This care is particularly important when the recommended agent is a new or infrequently used drug.

99 00 01 02 03/9 8 7 6 5 4 3 2 1

Contributors

Robert K. Bush, MD, FACP
Professor of Medicine (CHS)
University of Wisconsin-Madison;
Chief of Allergy
William S. Middleton VA Hospital
Madison, Wisconsin

William W. Busse, MD
Professor of Medicine
Head, Allergy and Immunology
Department of Medicine
University of Wisconsin Hospital and Clinics
Madison, Wisconsin

Hiroshi Chantaphakul, MD
Post-Doctoral Fellow
Division of Allergy and Immunology
Department of Medicine
University of Wisconsin Hospital and Clinics
Madison, Wisconsin

Ernest N. Charlesworth, MD, FACP
Department of Allergy and Dermatology
University of Texas Medical School
Houston, Texas;
Department of Allergy and Dermatology
Scott and White Clinic
College Station, Texas

Mark S. Dykewicz, MD
Associate Professor of Internal Medicine
Division of Allergy and Immunology
Saint Louis University School of Medicine
St. Louis, Missouri

Jordan N. Fink, MD
Professor of Medicine
Department of Medicine and Pediatrics;
Chief, Allergy and Immunology Division
Medical College of Wisconsin
Milwaukee, Wisconsin

Roger W. Fox, MD
Associate Professor of Medicine and Public
  Health
Division of Allergy and Immunology
Department of Occupational and
  Environmental Health
University of South Florida Health Sciences
  Center
James A. Haley Veterans Hospital
Tampa, Florida

Phil Lieberman, MD, FACP
Clinical Professor of Medicine and
  Pediatrics
Division of Allergy and Immunology
Department of Medicine and Pediatrics
University of Tennessee College of
  Medicine
Cordova, Tennessee

Richard F. Lockey, MD
Professor of Medicine, Pediatrics, and Public
  Health
Joy McCann Culverhouse Professor in
  Allergy and Immunology
University of South Florida College of
  Medicine;
Director, Division of Allergy and
  Immunology
James A. Haley Veterans' Hospital
Tampa, Florida

Robert P. Nelson, Jr., MD
Associate Professor of Medicine and
  Pediatrics
University of South Florida
All Children's Hospital
St. Petersburg, Florida

Robert E. Reisman, MD, MACP
Clinical Professor of Medicine and
  Pediatrics
State University of New York at Buffalo
Buffalo, New York

Raymond G. Slavin, MD, FACP
Professor of Internal Medicine and Molecular
  Microbiology and Immunology
Director, Division of Allergy and
  Immunology
Saint Louis University School of Medicine
St. Louis, Missouri

Michael C. Zacharisen, MD, FAAP
Assistant Professor of Medicine (Allergy) and
  Pediatrics
Department of Medicine and Pediatrics
Medical College of Wisconsin
Milwaukee, Wisconsin

Foreword

One of the slings and arrows of outrageous fortune is to inherit the genes that predispose us to allergic diseases. In the spring, instead of inhaling the glorious fragrances of the trees, grasses, and flowers, we rub our eyes, blow our noses, and try to catch our breaths. Our flesh is heir to rashes; to swelling of the eyes, throats, and larynges; and sometimes to life-threatening anaphylaxis. To add insult to injury, we often fail to get relief from countless nonprescription remedies. Although television advertisements hawk new, miraculous, nonsedating prescription drugs for our allergic ills, we often discover that our general internists are ill-prepared to give us solid advice about therapy. This lack of expertise is not surprising given 1) the short shrift medical schools give to allergic diseases, and 2) the general lack of allergy training in internal medicine training programs.

In *Expert Guide to Allergy and Immunology,* Drs. Raymond Slavin and Robert Reisman come to the rescue. Each of the editors of this valuable aid for general internists is a distinguished allergist who not only is steeped in fundamental research into the mechanisms of atopic response but also has decades of experience in the management of allergic diseases. Both have spent countless hours preventing and treating the discomforts and threats of seasonal rhinitis, asthma, eczema, insect allergies, and life-threatening allergic emergencies.

In the interest of full disclosure, I feel a little like the book's godfather. Some years ago, I chaired the American College of Physicians' Scientific Program subcommittee–the group charged with setting the agenda for the College's annual scientific teaching sessions. From my own experiences and those of my family and my patients, I was cognizant of the frequency, importance, and inexpert treatment of allergic diseases. So, I asked Dr. Reisman (who has been a close friend of mine for more than 50 years) to organize two workshops. Since then, he and Dr. Slavin have participated in the meeting every year, drawing increasingly larger crowds to their teaching sessions as our health care system began to focus on enlarging the role of general internists in primary care.

This book is designed to accomplish just what their teaching sessions have done for years, i.e., give solid, scientifically based advice to physicians who are trying to give comfort to those who wheeze, sneeze, and suffer the ravages of allergic disease. I predict this will be one of those books that general internists wear out with repeated use.

Jerome P. Kassirer, MD, MACP
Editor-in-Chief
New England Journal of Medicine

Preface

The idea for this book grew out of a series of workshops addressing common allergic problems encountered by the internist that we gave at annual meetings of the American College of Physicians. We were impressed not only with the general interest of the registrants but also with the wide range of questions and comments—from the basic to the sophisticated.

Despite the fact that allergic diseases are the most common group of chronic medical disorders that occur in the United States, approximately half of the medical schools in the country have no full-time allergists. It is evident that the subject is not adequately taught in many schools and in many internal medicine residency programs. We felt, therefore, that there was a significant need for this book, and we have designed it with the primary care internist in mind. Our charge to the authors was to make it readable, concise, and eminently practical. We wanted to stress efficient, cost-effective approaches to diagnosis and management. As a way of bringing the material into the office setting, this book features illustrative case histories—a technique that was well received in our annual meeting workshops.

The subject material includes the usual allergic conditions likely to be seen by the primary care internist, namely allergic rhinitis, bronchial asthma, and allergic skin diseases. Diagnostic testing and immunotherapy are two topics commonly misunderstood by primary care physicians, and we thought it important to put these subjects in context. Thirty-five million people in the United States have sinusitis, and because it is frequently seen as a complication of allergic rhinitis, we decided to include this subject as well. Generally, the most serious of the allergic diseases—anaphylaxis—is seen first by the primary care physician, and we thought it vital to convey the proper approach to diagnosis, management, and appropriate referral. The remaining three subjects—drug reactions, immunologic lung diseases, and immunodeficiencies—are woefully ignored in most internal medicine training programs and yet all three conditions are generally seen first by the primary care physician.

After deciding on the subjects to be covered, our next task was to choose appropriate authors. We felt they should be 1) certified in internal medicine, 2) members of internal medicine departments, and, most importantly, 3) in touch with the needs of the practicing internist. We think the reader will agree that we have chosen wisely and that each author has answered his charge extremely well.

We are grateful to the American College of Physicians for affording us the opportunity to participate in this unique and ultimately satisfying endeavor. We particularly express our thanks to Mary Ruff for her unflagging enthusiasm and encouragement.

Raymond G. Slavin, MD, FACP
Robert E. Reisman, MD, MACP

Contents

Chapter 1

Diagnostic Tests in Allergy

Robert K. Bush, MD

Introduction

Scope of Allergic Diseases

Allergic diseases are common clinical problems. More than 50 million people in the United States suffer from allergic rhinitis, making it the most common chronic disease of both adults and children (1). Asthma, which affects 20 to 30 million people in the United States, also has, in many instances, an allergic basis involved in its pathogenesis (1). Anaphylactic reactions to foods, drugs, and insect stings along with allergic skin conditions, such as atopic dermatitis and urticaria, affect additional numbers of patients. Recognition of the factors that are involved in these reactions can reduce the morbidity and mortality of the diseases as well as the costs of treatment.

Mechanism of the Allergic Response

Allergic diseases arise from genetic and environmental factors. Allergic diseases, such as allergic rhinitis, asthma, and eczema, are often familial. The term *atopic disease* has been coined to describe these conditions. Although the genetics of allergic diseases are not completely understood, intensive investigations are underway to identify the genetic basis of these conditions. Exposure of the susceptible host to environmental allergens (proteins, glycoproteins) results in the production of IgE antibodies. Allergens are taken up by antigen-presenting cells, such as macrophages, and are presented to CD4+ T-helper lymphocytes. The T-helper cells interact with B cells, which under the influence of cytokines such as IL-4 and IL-5 lead to the production of specific IgE antibodies by mature plasma cells. The specific IgE antibodies circulate and attach to mast cells and basophils via the receptors for the Fc portion of the IgE molecule. Mast cells are found in abundance in the conjunctiva, nasal mucosa, lower respiratory tract, gastrointestinal tract, and skin. Once the individual has become sensitized (i.e., develops IgE antibodies), re-exposure to the allergen leads to the release of histamine, prostaglandins, leukotrienes, and other mediators from mast cells and basophils via the bridging by the antigen of antigen-specific IgE molecules on the surface of these cells. The chemical mediators result in vasodilation, smooth-muscle constriction, increased mucus secretion, and pruritus. These effects occur within minutes after exposure to the allergen, thus earning the term *immediate hypersensitivity*. In addition, an inflammatory component to the IgE-mediated reaction is well established. This response typically occurs at 3 to 5 hours, reaches a peak between 6 and 12 hours, and resolves within 24 hours; it has been termed the *late-phase response*. This reaction is characterized by the influx of basophils and eosinophils as well as other inflammatory cells into the site. It has been observed in the skin, nose, lung, and in systemic anaphylactic reactions; thus, allergic diseases represent the culmination of a series of immunologic and biochemical events.

The Role of Diagnostic Tests in Allergic Diseases

History and physical examination are essential in the diagnosis of any condition, including allergic diseases. A selection of cost-effective diagnostic tests assists the physician in confirming the clinical impression.

A variety of tests have been developed that examine various components of the allergic response. Measurements of total serum IgE levels, detection of specific IgE antibodies, measurement of biochemical mediators, and examination of tissues and secretions for eosinophils assist the clinician in the diagnosis. In some instances, a provocative challenge with the suspected allergen (e.g., an oral challenge with aspirin in the aspirin-sensitive asthmatic or a double-blind, placebo-controlled food challenge in the case of food-induced anaphylaxis) is necessary. The use of these various diagnostic tests is discussed in this chapter and in Chapters 2, 4, 5, 6, and 7.

For many allergic diseases, the demonstration of the presence of specific IgE antibodies by in vivo methods (skin testing) or in vitro methods is the most useful. This chapter concentrates on these diagnostic tools but touches on other methods as well.

Case 1.1

A 25-year-old nonsmoking graduate student recently moved into a ground-floor apartment in November. He had a history of childhood asthma that previously had been easily managed by the use of inhaled β-agonist as needed. Within 1 month of moving into his new apartment, he began to experience nocturnal awakenings, decreased exercise tolerance, and increased need for his β-agonist medication.

Physical examination revealed a pale, boggy nasal mucosa and scattered expiratory wheezes on auscultation of the chest.

Spirometry revealed a forced expiratory volume in 1 second (FEV_1) of 70% of predicted normal value and a forced vital capacity (FVC) of 98% of predicted normal value.

Following administration of β-agonist, there was improvement in FEV_1 to 90% of predicted normal value. Prick skin testing to inhalant allergens revealed 4+ reaction to house dust mite, 2+ to ragweed pollen, and 2+ to tree pollen.

The patient was treated with inhaled corticosteroids and instructed in environmental control measures to reduce exposure to house dust mites. After 3 months, the patient's pulmonary symptoms had improved. His FEV_1 was 95% of predicted normal value, with no significant response following bronchodilator therapy, and he had returned to only occasional use of the β-agonist inhaler. After an additional 2 months, the inhaled corticosteroid was withdrawn, and the patient continued to do well.

This case illustrates the importance of identifying specific allergenic responses. The elimination of an environmental factor (in this case, the house–dust-mite allergen) resulted in clinical improvement as well as decreased health care costs.

In Vivo Detection of Specific IgE Antibodies

Skin Testing

Indications
Skin tests for the detection of specific IgE antibodies to inhalant, food, drug, and venom allergens are the most widely used for the diagnosis of allergy because of their simplicity, rapidity of results, low cost, and high sensitivity (Box 1.1) (1–5). Selection of appropriate allergens for testing obviously will depend on the clinical disease. For allergic rhinitis and asthma, inhalant allergens are appropriate because food allergens rarely, if ever, cause rhinitis or asthma symptoms. In cases of suspected drug allergy, testing to medication, such as penicillin, and local anesthetics may be indicated. (This is discussed more fully in Chapter 7.) Likewise, anaphylactic reactions to suspected foods or stinging insects can be tested (*see* Chapter 6).

Box 1.1 Indications and Contraindications for Allergen Skin Testing

Indications	Contraindications
Inhalant sensitivity	*Absolute*
Allergic rhinitis	Inability to discontinue antihistamines
Asthma	Generalized skin disease
Food sensitivity	*Relative*
Atopic dermatitis	Pregnancy
Urticaria	β-Adrenergic–receptor blocking
Anaphylaxis	agent therapy
Drug reactions	History of anaphylaxis to previous
Penicillin sensitivity	skin tests
Local anesthetic reactions	Dermatographism
Stinging-insect anaphylaxis	Unstable angina

Adapted with permission from Bush RK, Gern JE. Allergy evaluation: who, what and how. In: Schidlow DV, Smith D, eds. A Practitioner's Guide to Pediatric Respiratory Disorders. Philadelphia: Hanley & Belfus; 1994:261–70.

In patients presenting with rhinitis symptoms, whether on a seasonal or perennial basis, appropriate skin allergen testing can identify the suspected allergens. In patients with asthma, skin testing for inhalant allergens allows for the identification of the relevant exposure. Such knowledge can be useful in making recommendations in terms of environmental control measures or appropriate immunotherapy.

Evaluation of Patients Before Skin Testing

Before skin testing, the patient must be evaluated by an experienced physician who is familiar with the nuances of skin testing (4). This evaluation is not only necessary to establish that the patient's condition is likely to have an allergic basis but also to evaluate the patient for possible risks to skin testing (Boxes 1.2 and 1.3).

Although skin testing using epicutaneous (prick/puncture) methods is generally safe, there is always a risk of a systemic anaphylactic reaction; therefore, a physician experienced in treating anaphylactic reactions must always be present and available during skin testing. Necessary equipment for treating systemic anaphylaxis (e.g., epinephrine, intravenous solutions for volume expansion, and equipment and supplies for airway protection) should be readily available. Because the effect of epinephrine may be blunted by the presence of β-blocker therapy, such medications should be discontinued before skin testing (4). Pregnancy is a relative contraindication to skin testing be-

---

Box 1.2 Factors Affecting Skin Test Response

Age of patient
Specific IgE titer
Test site: upper back more reactive than forearm
Quality of extracts: no standardized reagents for many allergens
Presence of dermatographism
Use of medications

Antihistamines inhibit skin test response for variable periods
   Astemizole: 60 days
   Hydroxyzine: 3 days
   Other antihistamines: 3 days
   Tricyclic antidepressants: 5 days
Prolonged use of topical corticosteroids may blunt response

Test technique
Prick more specific
Intradermal more sensitive

Reprinted with permission from Bush RK, Gern JE. Allergy evaluation: who, what and how. In: Schidlow DV, Smith D, eds. A Practitioner's Guide to Pediatric Respiratory Disorders. Philadelphia: Hanley & Belfus; 1994:261–70.

---

cause systemic anaphylaxis may produce hypoxemia in the fetus (4). Patients with severe lung disease, congestive heart failure, or unstable angina may not be appropriate candidates for skin testing because anaphylaxis is particularly likely to be life threatening in patients with limited cardiovascular reserve (4). Patients with severe allergic symptoms, particularly unstable asthma, should not be tested until their symptoms have been stabilized (4).

In addition, certain situations may invalidate the skin testing results. An area of normal skin must be available for testing; therefore, patients with extensive dermatitis are not appropriate candidates. Patients should not be taking antihistamine drugs or other medications that can attenuate the skin test response. Patients with marked dermatographism cannot be reliably tested. Following viral exanthema or sunburns, the skin may not be normally reactive for several weeks.

Epicutaneous Skin Testing

Prick tests have become the accepted screening method for detecting specific IgE antibodies in vivo (Box 1.4) (1,4,5). Scratch tests, which have been used in the past, are less reproducible than the prick method and are no longer used. The prick test is widely accepted because it is quicker and less painful,

---

Box 1.3 Approaches and Precautions for Skin Testing

Approaches

Select high quality extracts of appropriate concentrations.

Include positive and negative controls.

Perform tests on normal skin; evaluate for dermatographism.

Record results at proper time (10–15 min).

Precautions

Skin tests should never be performed unless a physician is immediately available to treat untoward reactions.

Emergency equipment and medications should be available.

Do not conduct testing if patient is experiencing marked symptoms.

Be aware of patient's current medications, i.e., β-blockers (increase severity of anaphylaxis), antihistamines (blunt skin test response).

Reprinted with permission from Bush RK, Gern JE. Allergy evaluation: who, what and how. In: Schidlow DV, Smith D, eds. A Practitioner's Guide to Pediatric Respiratory Disorders. Philadelphia: Hanley & Belfus; 1994:261–70.

---

has better specificity, is less likely to cause systemic reactions, and is less expensive than intradermal testing. This method has also been found to correlate better with clinical sensitivity. This, in part, may be due to the use of more stable reagents.

The prick test is performed on cleansed skin by passing a small needle through a drop of the allergenic extract at an approximate 45° angle to skin (Box 1.5) (5,6). The needle is pressed lightly into the epidermis, and the tip is gently lifted up to produce a pricking sensation. The skin prick should not be deep enough to produce visible bleeding. Another method is the puncture technique. A drop of allergenic extract is placed on the skin, and a puncture device is pushed into the skin perpendicularly. Commonly used puncture devices have a small point that penetrates approximately 1.0 to 1.5 mm into the skin. A bifurcated needle can also be used. The needle is pressed firmly against the skin through a drop of extract, and the needle is rocked back and forth or side to side.

A number of devices for performing prick skin tests are available. Metal needles generally give better reproducibility than plastic needles. Also used are hypodermic needles of 25–27 gauge and blood lancets. Multiple test devices (e.g., Multi-Test II), which use the puncture technique, have also been studied (7). It has been recommended that each skin testing laboratory establish criteria for positive and negative tests for whichever device is used (7).

Box 1.4 Selection of Skin Test Method

Prick skin tests are more specific than intradermal testing (i.e., fewer false positives).

Intradermal tests are more sensitive than prick method (i.e., fewer false negatives).

Prick skin testing should precede intradermal testing to decrease risk of anaphylactic reactions.

Prick skin tests are simple, rapid, and inexpensive.

Prick skin tests usually produce little discomfort.

Intradermal tests may be more reproducible.

Reprinted with permission from Bush RK, Gern JE. Allergy evaluation: who, what and how. In: Schidlow DV, Smith D, eds. A Practitioner's Guide to Pediatric Respiratory Disorders. Philadelphia: Hanley & Belfus; 1994:261–70.

Box 1.5 Procedure for Prick Skin Test

Devices
  25–27 gauge needles, blood lancets, multitest devices, bifurcated needles
Extracts
  1:10–1:20 weight:volume in 50% glycerine
Controls
  Histamine base 1 mg/mL
Diluent
  Number of tests for inhalants: 30–50

Reprinted with permission from Bush RK, Gern JE. Allergy evaluation: who, what and how. In: Schidlow DV, Smith D, eds. A Practitioner's Guide to Pediatric Respiratory Disorders. Philadelphia: Hanley & Belfus; 1994:261–70.

Using separate needles for each test is recommended, because wiping may not completely remove the allergenic extract from the tip of the needle and may additionally pose the risk of injury to the operator.

Allergenic extracts used for prick skin testing usually are prepared as 1:10 to 1:20 (weight:volume ratio) extracts stabilized in 50% glycerin (6). To preserve potency of extracts, they should be stored at 4°C until used and then returned immediately to a refrigerator (6). Appropriate controls consist of 1 mg/mL histamine base for a positive control (4,6). Others favor 9% codeine solution in 50% glycerin as a control (codeine stimulates direct mast cell degranulation) (6). A negative control, consisting of the diluent (e.g., phosphate-buffered saline solution at pH 7.4 with 0.4% phenol and 50% glycerin), is also applied (6).

For inhalant allergy testing, fewer than 30 skin tests are usually sufficient. There is seldom the need for more than 50 skin tests. Because specific IgE antibody to inhalant allergens rarely develop below the age of 2 years, skin testing in young patients for inhalant allergens is seldom indicated.

Interpretation: After pricking the skin, the extract is left on for 1 minute and then wiped off. The histamine-control effect will peak at approximately 10 minutes after application, whereas the allergens will peak at approximately 15 to 20 minutes. The largest and smallest diameters at right angles are added and then divided by two to obtain the dimensions of the wheal and of the surrounding erythema or "flare" response. Permanent records can be achieved by outlining the area of the erythema and wheal diameter using a pen, blotting it onto cellophane tape, and storing it on paper as part of the permanent record.

Various methods have been used to interpret skin test results (8). Most reactions indicative of clinical allergy are wheals greater than 3 mm in diameter. Grading is on a scale of 0 to 4; however, a higher grade does not necessarily indicate a higher degree of clinical symptoms (Table 1.1).

Errors in Performing Prick Skin Tests: Common errors resulting in erroneous skin test results include the following:

1. Placing skin test sites too close together (i.e., less than 2 cm apart).

Table 1.1 Interpretation of Skin Test Results

Prick		Intradermal		
Grade	Wheal	Grade	Wheal (mm)	Erythema (mm)
0	≤ Negative control	0	< 5	< 5
1	1 mm > control	±	5–10	5–10
2	2–4 mm > control	1	5–10	11–20
3	5 mm > control	2	5–10	21–30
4	Wheal with pseudopods	3	5–10 or with pseudopods	31–40
		4	> 15 or with many pseudopods	> 40

Reprinted with permission from Bush RK, Gern JE. Allergy evaluation: who, what and how. In: Schidlow DV, Smith D, eds. A Practitioner's Guide to Pediatric Respiratory Disorders. Philadelphia: Hanley & Belfus; 1994:261–70.

2. Bleeding at the site, resulting in false-negative reactions.
3. Insufficient cleansing (if wiping is used to clean needles) resulting in spreading of allergenic solutions and false-positive reactions.
4. Insufficient penetration of the skin (particularly with use of plastic devices) resulting in false-negative reactions.

With prick skin testing, the coefficient of variation is approximately 8% to 30% (6). With skilled operators using similar techniques, these margins of error can be reduced significantly. There is an approximate 5% false-negative rate of prick/puncture testing (6).

Intradermal Skin Testing

Indications: With the exception of skin testing for drug allergies and stinging-insect venoms, intradermal testing should be performed only after negative prick skin tests have been obtained to the allergen and a specific sensitivity is still suspected (4–6). Intradermal testing is not appropriate for food allergens because of a high degree of false-positive results and the risk of anaphylaxis. Intradermal skin testing, therefore, is usually reserved for patients in whom there is a need for a higher degree of sensitivity of the test; however, there is a reduction in the specificity of the results (i.e., more false-positive reactions).

Method: Unitized 0.5- to 1.0-mL hubless syringes with a 26–30-gauge needle should be employed for intradermal skin testing (Box 1.6) (6). The syringes should be discarded after each use because of possible contamination by infectious agents. For intradermal use, stock allergenic extracts are diluted to the appropriate concentration with 0.03% human serum albumin–saline solution (6). The volume injected into the skin is 0.01 to 0.05 mL. The bevel of the needle should always be directed downward. This assures contact of the allergen with the underlying mast cells and avoids splashing in the eyes of the operator. The concentration of the allergenic extracts should be between 10 and 1000 allergy units (AU)/mL (1:100 to 1:1000 weight:volume) (6). Appropriate positive controls consist of histamine (0.1 mg/mL) or codeine phosphate and the diluent as a negative control (6). The number of tests usually should not exceed 30.

Interpretation: Following injection of the allergen into the skin, readings are made at approximately 15 to 20 minutes. Measurements of the wheal and flare diameter in two directions are averaged as with prick skin tests. As concentration of the allergens is increased, the frequency of positive results increases. Glycerin-stabilized allergens should be avoided because they may give false-positive results. The coefficient of variation with intradermal skin testing is approximately 5% to 17% (6). A number of grading systems for intradermal skin testing have been proposed; one of the more commonly used

---

Box 1.6 Intradermal Skin Test Technique

Devices

Unitized 0.5–1.0 mL hubless syringes with 26–30 gauge needles, disposable after one-time use

Extracts

Diluted with 0.3% human serum albumin–saline at 1:100–1:1000 weight:volume (1000 protein nitrogen units/10–1000 allergen units/mL)

Volume injected

0.01–0.05 mL

Controls

Histamine base at 0.1 mg/mL or codeine phosphate

Diluent

Number of tests

For inhalants: up to 30 tests

Not appropriate for food allergens

Reprinted with permission from Bush RK, Gern JE. Allergy evaluation: who, what and how. In: Schidlow DV, Smith D, eds. A Practitioner's Guide to Pediatric Respiratory Disorders. Philadelphia: Hanley & Belfus; 1994:261–70.

---

is that recommended by Norman (8) (*see* Table 1.1). A grading scale of 0 to 4 is used based on the wheal and erythema. A localized wheal without erythema is usually clinically insignificant.

Errors: Errors in intradermal skin testing include the following:

1. The skin test sites are too close together (< 2 cm), resulting in false-positive reactions.
2. The volume injected into the skin is too large (> 0.05 mL), resulting in false-positive reactions.
3. High concentrations of allergens, resulting in false-positive reactions.
4. Injection of air into the skin, leading to the so-called "splash" reactions and causing false-positive reactions.
5. Presence of intracutaneous bleeding interpreted as a positive reaction.
6. Subcutaneous injection of the allergen, producing a false-negative reaction.
7. Although the risk of systemic reactions is low, a negative skin test result to the allergen in question should be obtained before proceeding to intradermal testing.

8. Application of too many tests at once may lead to systemic reactions in sensitive patients.
9. In all situations, a positive skin test result must be correlated with a patient's history (1,4).

It has been shown that the presence of positive intradermal skin tests alone does not indicate clinical sensitivity in subjects with negative prick skin tests.

Factors Influencing Skin Tests

The area of the body into which the skin test is applied will affect results (*see* Box 1.2) (1,4). The middle and upper back are more reactive than the lower part of the back. Likewise, the skin of the back is more reactive than the forearm. The volar surface of the forearm is often chosen as a skin test site because it is readily accessible. Skin tests should be placed in the middle area of the forearm, because the antecubital fossa is more reactive than the wrist area. The ulnar side of the forearm is more reactive than the radial side. Because of overlap between reaction sites, the extracts should be placed at least 2 to 4 cm apart.

The age of the patient will also influence the skin test reactivity. Infants may often show large erythematous flares compared with adults (1,4). The size of the skin test reaction increases from infancy to adulthood but declines after approximately 50 years of age.

Pathologic conditions can also affect the skin test reactivity. For example, skin test reactivity is decreased in patients undergoing chronic hemodialysis, in patients with peripheral neuropathy, and in patients with malignancies.

Clearly, the use of antihistamine medications can influence skin test results (1,4). Use of H_1 antihistamines, such as astemizole, must be stopped at least 60 days before skin testing. Hydroxyzine must be stopped for at least 72 hours, and nonsedating, newer antihistamines (e.g., cetirizine, loratadine, and fexofenadine) need to be stopped at least 3 days before testing. H_2 blockers, tricyclic antidepressants, some phenothiazine preparations, and prolonged use of topical corticosteroids may also diminish skin test reactivity.

Safety of Skin Testing

As previously mentioned, skin testing should not be conducted in patients who are receiving β-blocker therapy (6). Likewise, pregnancy is a relative contraindication (6). Patients with severe cardiovascular pulmonary disease and those with active allergic symptoms, such as unstable asthma, should not be skin tested (6).

The risk of an adverse reaction to prick skin testing is approximately 0.04% for systemic reactions. There have been no reports of fatalities. With intradermal testing, systemic reactions occur in approximately 1% to 2% of patients, and deaths have been reported (6). These primarily occurred in patients who had not undergone previous prick skin testing.

Specific Allergens for Testing

In selecting allergens for testing, several factors should be considered. The first consideration is whether identification of the allergens will improve the quality of the patient's care either by the institution of specific avoidance measures or by immunotherapy. Secondly, allergen testing may also be used as a predictor of when a patient's symptoms may worsen so that medical therapy can be escalated at appropriate times. Thirdly, specific allergens used in the testing depend on the nature of those found in the area where the patient resides. Pollens from trees, grasses, and weeds vary in different portions of the United States, and knowledge of the botany of the area in which the patient resides is useful in determining which materials to select for testing. Lastly, the availability of suitable extracts for testing should be considered. Currently, in the United States, only a limited number of allergens have been standardized for composition and concentration of the relevant allergens.

House Dust Mites

Because sensitivity to house dust mites is a major cause of allergic respiratory disease and is linked with the development of asthma, it is important to identify this allergen. The two major species of house dust mite in the United States are *Dermatophagoides pteronyssinus* and *D. farinae*. Standardized allergenic extracts of these are available for testing.

Animal Danders

Large numbers of patients are exposed to domestic cats. Sensitivity to cat dander has been linked to the development of asthma in children. The major allergen responsible for cat sensitivity is the protein Fel d 1. Two principle forms of cat allergen extracts are available: an epithelial-derived preparation that contains mainly Fel d 1 and a cat pelt extract that contains both Fel d 1 and albumin. Some patients are sensitive to the cat albumin. A patient whose test results are negative to the epithelial-derived preparation may react to the cat-pelt extract. Both extracts contain adequate amounts of the Fel d 1 to detect the most sensitive individuals.

Sensitivity to dog dander is somewhat less common than sensitivity to cats. The major allergens responsible for dog allergy are not as well characterized as those for cat allergy, although the protein Can f 1 has been identified. Currently available extracts in the United States are not standardized and, therefore, are subject to significant variability.

Testing may be conducted to extracts from rabbits, hamsters, gerbils, rats, and mice for patients who are exposed to these animals either as pets or occupationally. The extracts are not standardized.

Grass

Grass pollens are among the most common cause of allergy world wide and affect an estimated 10% to 30% of allergic patients. A number of species of grass have been implicated in allergic disease. Kentucky blue grass, rye, timothy, red top, and sweet vernal grass are among the more common varieties. In certain portions of the United States, other species of grasses, such as Bermuda and Johnson grass, may be important. The allergenic components of most grass species are extensively cross-reactive; however, Bermuda and Johnson grass may contain unique allergenic components. In general, mixtures of grass-pollen extracts will identify patients with sensitivity to grass pollen, and testing for individual grass pollens is seldom needed. Standardized extracts are now available.

Trees

Tree species responsible for allergic disease vary according to the geographic location. Most important tree pollens in North America arise from deciduous trees, including birch, beech, oak, maple, elm, willow, poplar, aspen, olive, and ash. The mountain cedar tree, found in Texas and parts of the Southwestern United States, also accounts for seasonal allergic rhinitis and asthma. Extracts of standardized tree pollen extracts are not available in the United States. Selection of appropriate testing material depends on the expertise of the physician.

Weeds

The major weed pollen in the United States is ragweed. Two important species are short ragweed (*Ambrosia artemisiaefolia*) and giant ragweed (*A. trifida*), although other species are found at different locations. Other weeds that cause difficulty include the Amaranths and Chenopods. Weed pollens appear to be extensively cross-reactive, although some possess unique antigens. Standardized extracts of ragweed have been available for a number of years; however, other weed pollens have not been standardized to date.

Fungi

An extensive number of fungi are allergenic. Unfortunately, the complexity of these allergens has prevented the availability of standardized extracts. Many of the extracts are of poor quality. The most important fungus is *Alternaria*, which has been linked to the development of asthma and to severe and fatal asthma attacks. *Cladosporium*, *Aspergillus*, and *Penicillium* are also important fungal allergens. A variety of other species may contribute to allergen exposure, but their overall significance is not completely understood. Species of *Basidiomycetes* may be important in certain locations, but no commercially available extracts are available.

Insects

A growing body of evidence suggests that in inner city areas cockroach allergy may be an important precipitant of asthma. Skin test reactivity to extracts of cockroaches has been found in asthmatic children. No standardized extracts of cockroach allergens are available.

Food

Food allergy is seldom a cause of isolated respiratory symptoms, but it may be considered in young infants who have respiratory difficulties after ingestion of milk or other foods. No food extracts are standardized; therefore, their potency and quality are questionable. In some instances, a prick skin test after direct application to the skin of fresh fruits and vegetables may be useful. Food-allergy testing is appropriate in cases of urticaria, anaphylaxis, and eczema. These are discussed in further detail in Chapter 5.

Drugs

Skin testing is available for certain drugs, such as penicillin. Their clinical use is discussed in Chapter 7.

Venoms

For cases of anaphylaxis due to stinging-insect venoms, appropriate skin tests are available. This is discussed in detail in Chapter 6.

In Vitro Assays for Specific IgE Antibodies

Indications for Measurement of Specific IgE Antibodies by In Vitro Tests

In some instances, skin testing may not be possible. Patients who are unable to discontinue antihistamine therapy before skin testing may be candidates for in vitro testing (Box 1.7) (2,3,6,9,10). Patients who have extensive dermatitis or dermatographism may not be able to undergo appropriate skin testing

---

Box 1.7 Specific IgE In Vitro Tests

Patients unable to discontinue antihistamines
Patients with extensive dermatitis/dermatographia
Patients unable to discontinue beta-blockers
Patients with an anaphylactic sensitivity to foods

(6,9,10). Patients who are unable to discontinue β-blocker therapy are candidates for in vitro testing (6,9,10). For patients who have had severe anaphylactic reactions to foods in which the risk of skin tests may lead to an adverse reaction, in vitro testing may be performed (6,9,10).

Methods

A number of systems for the detection of allergen-specific IgE antibodies are available (9,10). One of the most commonly used systems is based on the principle of immunoabsorption. The specific allergen is bound to a solid phase support (sorbent). The patient's serum is added. If antibodies specific for the allergen are present, they are detected by an enzyme-linked or radiolabeled antihuman IgE antibody. The quantity of anti-IgE bound to the solid phase is measured and expressed as either units of specific IgE or as a class score. The earliest of these tests was called the *radioallergosorbent test* (RAST). These assays are capable of detecting specific IgE antibodies in concentrations of nanograms per milliliter of serum.

Interpretation

Some laboratories report results by calculating the ratio of the test serum to the results of serum from nonallergic individuals tested in the same way. These are expressed as ratios, with a ratio of greater than or equal to 2.5 considered to be positive (9,10). Other laboratories reported results in class scores ranging from 0 to 5 (9,10). Class 0 would indicate a nondetectable level of IgE, whereas the increasing classes represent increasing quantities of IgE. To increase the sensitivity of in vitro assays, scoring systems have been modified. The modified scoring system produces an apparent increase in the sensitivity of the test at the expense of sensitivity, because only the scoring system, not the actual detection limit of assay, is changed. It is important to recognize that the results are semiquantitative and do not translate into clinical sensitivity.

The sensitivity and specificity in an in vitro test can vary markedly from one allergen to another. In some systems, sensitivities of 70% to 80% have been noted when compared with skin tests, whereas with other allergens a correlation of less than 50% has been noted (9,10). Appropriate in vitro tests correlate up to 70% to 80% of the time with prick skin tests, but sensitivity is not usually as high (9,10).

Advantages/Disadvantages of In Vitro Tests

In vitro tests are convenient for patients who may not have access to physicians trained in appropriate skin testing techniques. In vitro tests can be performed in patients receiving medications for which allergy skin testing would be contraindicated (1,4). The results are not dependent on the condition of the skin (1,4). There is no risk of anaphylaxis from in vitro testing (1,4).

On the other hand, in vitro testing is more expensive in general than skin testing for a similar number of allergens, and the availability of allergens is limited (4). It is not as sensitive as properly performed skin tests in most instances. There are time delays for in vitro results, whereas skin test results are available within 10 to 15 minutes of their application.

Cost Effectiveness

Prick skin testing is generally safe; however, reproducibility and interpretation are highly dependent on the skill and experience of the operator. Skin testing using the intradermal method exposes the patient to a small but real risk of an anaphylactic reaction. Although it is more sensitive than prick skin testing, the intradermal technique loses the specificity of the reaction. For this reason it may be better to refer patients for intradermal testing to an appropriate allergy/immunology specialist (1,4).

Because a large number of allergens can be evaluated by skin testing techniques at one time, the cost per test is much less than for in vitro testing. In vitro testing may be appropriate when skin testing cannot be performed appropriately or when there is risk of anaphylaxis to the patient (1,4,9,10).

Total IgE Level

Utility of Total IgE Measurement

Some physicians use total serum IgE levels to determine whether asthma or rhinitis have an allergic basis; however, due to the considerable overlap in total serum IgE levels among patients with asthma or other allergic disease and healthy individuals, the measurement of total serum IgE levels is of limited diagnostic utility. A more effective diagnostic test is the detection of specific IgE antibodies by skin test or in vitro methods with an appropriate panel of allergens as cited earlier (9,10).

In addition to asthma, allergic rhinitis, and eczema, a variety of conditions are associated with elevations of total IgE. These include parasitic infections, immunodeficiency states (e.g., hyper-IgE syndrome), malignancy (e.g., Hodgkin's disease), and autoimmune diseases. Although measurements of total IgE levels are not generally useful for the diagnosis of allergic disease, total serum IgE levels are valuable in the diagnosis and management of allergic bronchopulmonary aspergillosis (ABPA) (*see* chapter 8). Typically, patients with this condition have serum IgE levels of greater than 500 IU/mL. During the stage of ABPA in which pulmonary infiltrates are present, the total IgE level is usually markedly elevated; a normal total IgE level virtually excludes the diagnosis (9). With therapy of ABPA, the total IgE level tends to fall. A sudden increase in serum IgE level may herald an exacerbation and allow time for the physician to institute or increase corticosteroid therapy to prevent further lung damage.

Test Methods and Interpretation

A variety of methods have been developed to detect the small concentrations of IgE normally present in human serum (9,10). The most commonly used methods employ a two-site immunoassay using monoclonal antihuman IgE antibodies (4,9,10). The results of the IgE measurement are generally expressed as international units (IU) per milliliter (mL). One IU equals 2.4 ng of protein. More recently, the SI unit has been adopted. One SI unit equals 1 µg/L of protein. Most commercially available assays are accurate to concentrations of less than 5 IU/mL (12 ng/mL) of IgE (4,9,10). The concentration of IgE in serum is highly age dependent (9,10). Mean serum IgE levels increase in normal children to approximately 10 to 15 years of age. There is an age-dependent decline in the second through eighth decade of life.

Most studies have shown that the total serum IgE concentrations tend to be higher in allergic adults and children compared with nonallergic individuals of similar age (9,10). There is, however, a large degree of overlap between serum IgE concentrations in allergic and nonallergic individuals, which limits the diagnostic value of the test (9,10). After 14 years of age, serum IgE values greater than 333 IU/mL are considered to be elevated. If a high value of IgE is chosen to distinguish allergic from nonallergic individuals, the specificity of the tests is often greater than 90%, but the sensitivity is low at 30% to 50% (9,10). Age-specific elevation of total IgE levels has been identified as a risk factor for asthma; however, a low or normal IgE level does not eliminate the possibility of allergic mechanisms (9,10).

Other Tests

Measurement of Chemical Mediators

Tryptase

Tryptase is a protein produced by mast cells. Unlike histamine, it is stable in biologic fluids (11). Serum β-tryptase has been found to be a useful marker for the diagnosis of systemic anaphylaxis. Elevated levels of β-tryptase can be found up to 2 hours following the event. For unexplained episodes of hypotension or syncope, it may be useful to obtain a β-tryptase level if mast cell activation is suspected. Normal serum β-tryptase levels are less than 1 ng/mL.

Plasma and Urinary Histamine Levels

Urinary histamine levels may be a possible marker for anaphylaxis and also for the diagnosis of systemic mastocytosis. The levels can be quite variable and are influenced by the presence of bacteria in the urine. A major metabolite of histamine, 1,4-methylimidiazole-4 acidic acid, has been shown to be useful in the diagnosis of systemic mastocytosis, but its availability is limited. Plasma histamine levels have also been suggested as a marker for mast cell activation, but its measurement is difficult. Fluorometric and radioenzymatic methods that have detection limits as low as 10 pg/mL are available; however, the routine, clinical use of these measurements has yet to be shown effective (11).

Other Mast Cell Mediators

Prostaglandin D_2 is a marker for mast cell activation. This prostaglandin is produced by mast cells, not by basophils. It can be measured in secretions and urine. Increased levels of prostaglandin D_2 have been found in the urine of patients with systemic mastocytosis (11). Similarly, α-protryptase has been shown to be elevated in the serum of patients with systemic mastocytosis. Neither test is available commercially (11).

Leukotriene E_4 is an arachidonic acid metabolite produced by many cells. Measurement of leukotriene E_4 levels are primarily used for research purposes. Increased urinary leukotriene E_4 have been demonstrated following bronchospastic reactions to aspirin in aspirin-sensitive asthmatics as well as after allergen-induced bronchoconstriction that follows bronchoprovocation challenge (11).

Peripheral Blood Eosinophil Counts

Elevation of the peripheral blood eosinophil count is suggestive but not diagnostic of allergic disease. Approximately 30% to 40% of patients with allergic rhinitis and asthma may demonstrate peripheral blood eosinophilia. It should be noted that patients with asthma may have elevation of the peripheral blood eosinophil count even though there is no evidence for an allergic component to their disease. Total peripheral blood eosinophil counts, therefore, are of limited value in the diagnosis of allergic diseases. A variety of causes for peripheral blood eosinophilia are known; however, peripheral blood eosinophil counts have been shown to be inversely related to the FEV_1 in patients with asthma (i.e., the higher the total peripheral blood eosinophil count, the lower the FEV_1). Peripheral blood eosinophilia can be a marker for patients who may have a reversible component to obstructive airway disease, and there is an association between the degree of eosinophilia and the severity of asthma.

Nasal and Sputum Eosinophilia

A nasal smear for eosinophils is sometimes useful in evaluating patients with allergic rhinitis. During active allergic rhinitis, the eosinophil count may comprise up to 25% of the total cell count. On the other hand, patients with the nonallergic rhinitis with eosinophilia syndrome (which is an entity of unknown etiology) also have eosinophils in nasal secretions. To the best of our knowledge, this is not an IgE-mediated condition. The presence of a preponderance of neutrophils suggests the presence of an infectious process (e.g., viral upper respiratory tract infection or bacterial sinusitis).

The technique for obtaining nasal secretions for eosinophils consists of having the individual blow his or her nose into wax paper, smearing the secretions on a glass slide, air drying the slide, and then staining for eosinophils using Giemsa or Wright's stain. The slide is then examined under light microscopy, and the total number of eosinophils is determined.

Sputum eosinophilia often occurs in active asthma; however, the diagnostic utility is limited. It is not necessarily reflective of an allergic etiology, because sputum eosinophilia can occur in patients with nonallergic asthma.

Provocation Testing

On rare occasions, it may be necessary to refer a patient to an appropriate specialist for provocation testing. This may include conjunctival challenge, nasal challenge, or bronchoprovocation in instances when an allergic reaction cannot be demonstrated by other techniques (12).

Bronchoprovocation challenges for asthma are not indicated as a routine diagnostic procedure. In some instances, such as an occupational exposure, they may be necessary to establish the diagnosis (4,12). Testing should be done only by experienced specialists. The patient must have stable pulmonary function with an FEV_1 of at least 80% of predicted normal value. Medications that interfere with the results of the tests (e.g., cromolyn, antihistamines, and inhaled β-agonists) are withheld before the challenge. The patient inhales saline, and the pulmonary functions are repeated. If the baseline FEV_1 remains stable, the patient inhales increasing doses of the challenge substance at 15- to 30-minute intervals. A decrease in FEV_1 of at least 20% following a dose of the substance is considered a positive response. Testing is terminated if this reduction is achieved, or it is continued until the maximal dose is given without a change in FEV_1 (negative challenge) (12).

Patients experiencing adverse reactions to foods may require further evaluation by appropriate provocative challenges (2). These consist of double-blind, placebo-controlled challenges using encapsulated food. Sequentially increasing doses of the suspected food are administered at intervals of 30 to 60 minutes until the patient consumes an amount equivalent to a standard serving size of the food in question. If the patient demonstrates objective evidence of an allergic reaction (e.g., urticaria, erythema, or flare of eczema) or other adverse reaction, then the procedure is halted and appropriate therapy administered. The tests are conducted on separate days, using placebo on one occasion and the challenge food on the other. Both the person administering the challenge capsules and the patient are blinded to the contents, and only after the test is completed are the identities revealed. Such testing is rarely indicated in the diagnosis of suspected food anaphylaxis because, in most instances, appropriate tests for specific IgE antibody can reveal the cause.

Basophil Histamine–Release Assays

By the use of density centrifugation, circulating basophils can be isolated from blood. The isolated cells can be challenged in vitro, using allergens to which the patient has specific IgE antibodies attached to the surface of the cells. The stimulation results in the release of histamine from the basophils, which can be measured by appropriate assays. The amount of histamine released by the allergen stimulus is compared with the total amount of histamine released after lysis of the cells. The results are then expressed as a percentage of histamine released. These tests are technically difficult to perform and have little, if any, clinical use (6).

Eosinophil Cationic Protein Measurements

Eosinophils are rich in granular proteins that may contribute to the inflammatory response of allergic diseases. One of these granular proteins (eosinophilic cationic protein [ECP]) has been identified recently, and immunoassays for its detection in serum and secretions have been developed. ECP levels in sputum have been suggested as a marker for airway inflammation and for monitoring response to asthma therapy; however, the clinical use of these measurements has not been fully established and they are largely used for research purposes.

Inappropriate Testing

Inappropriate skin tests include selection of nonallergic substances, such as tobacco smoke and facial tissue. Because dust mites are the major cause of sensitivity, house-dust extracts that contain a variety of allergen substances are no longer recommended.

The use of sublingual or intercutaneous provocation testing has not been shown to have any merit when subjected to rigorous scientific analysis (13).

The use of in vitro tests for food-specific IgG or IgG_4 assays has not proven to be of value. Likewise, detection of food antigen–antibody complexes has not proven useful. Evidence of lymphocyte activation (e.g., tritium uptake or IL-2 production) is not considered to be a valid assay. Basophil degranulation has not been shown to correlate with the presence of allergic disease. Similarly, cytotoxic food tests, applied kinesiology, electrodiagnosis, and analysis of urine or hair for minerals, vitamins, and amino acid content have no proven basis for the diagnosis of allergic diseases (13).

Conclusions and Recommendations

A number of diagnostic tests are available to the physician to assist in the diagnosis of allergic disease. Although some tests such as total IgE levels or peripheral blood eosinophilia are suggestive, they are not diagnostic. Measurement of chemical mediators has limited clinical use. The most useful tests for establishing appropriate diagnosis include the detection of specific IgE antibodies by in vivo or in vitro methods. Skin testing by the prick method is a safe, rapid, and economical method for detecting clinically relevant sensitivities. Intradermal testing may be used in patients who have negative prick tests but who have symptoms that suggest an allergic cause. In vitro tests should be reserved for patients who are unable to undergo skin testing or for whom skin testing is not readily available. In vitro tests may be useful but are much more expensive on a cost-per-test basis than appropriate skin testing. Identification of relevant allergic exposures and the demonstration of specific IgE antibodies can assist the physician in establishing a diagnosis as well as in recommending appropriate interventions, including environmental control measures and immunotherapy in selected patients.

REFERENCES

1. **Bush RK, Gern JE**. Allergy evaluation: who, what, and how. In: Schidlow DV, Smith D, eds. A Practitioner's Guide to Pediatric Respiratory Disorders. Philadelphia: Hanley & Belfus; 1994:261–70.

2. **Van Arsdel PP Jr, Larson EB**. Diagnostic tests for patients with suspected allergic disease. Ann Intern Med. 1989;110:304–12.

3. **American College of Physicians**. Allergy testing [Position Paper]. Ann Intern Med. 1989;110:317–20.

4. **Ownby DR.** Diagnostic tests in allergy. In: Lieberman P, Anderson J, eds. Allergic Diseases: Diagnosis and Treatment. Totowa, NJ: Humana Press; 1997:27–36.

5. **Bousquet J, Michel FB.** In vivo methods for study of allergy: skin tests, techniques, and interpretation. In: Middleton E Jr, Reed CE, Ellis EF, Adkinson NF Jr, Yunginger JW, Busse WW, eds. Allergy: Principles and Practice. 4th ed. St. Louis: CV Mosby; 1993:573–94.

6. **Bernstein IL.** Proceedings of the task force on guidelines for standardizing old and new technologies used for the diagnosis and treatment of allergic diseases. J Allergy Clin Immunol. 1988;82:487–526.

7. **Nelson HS, Lahr J, Buchmeier A, McCormick D.** Evaluation of devices for skin prick testing. J Allergy Clin Immunol. 1998;101:153–6.

8. **Norman PS.** Skin testing. In: Rose NR, de Macario EC, Fahey JL, Friedman H, Penn GM, eds. Manual of Clinical Laboratory Immunology. 4th ed. Washington, DC: American Society for Microbiology; 1992:685–8.

9. **Homburger HA, Katzmann JA.** Methods in laboratory immunology: principles and interpretation of laboratory tests for allergy. In: Middleton E Jr, Reed CE, Ellis EF, Adkinson NF Jr, Yunginger JW, Busse WW, eds. Allergy: Principles and Practice. 4th ed. St. Louis: CV Mosby; 1993:554–72.

10. **Hamilton RG, Adkinson NF Jr.** Assessment of human allergic diseases. In: Rich RR, Fleisher TA, Schwartz BD, Shearer WT, Strober W, eds. Clinical Immunology: Principles and Practice. St. Louis: CV Mosby; 1996:2169–86.

11. **Duff A, Schwartz LB.** Markers of mast cell degranulation. Methods. 1997;13:43–52.

12. **Peebles RS Jr, Hartert TV.** In vivo diagnostic procedures: skin testing, nasal provocation, and bronchial provocation. Methods. 1997;13:14–24.

13. **AAAI Training Program Directors' Committee.** A training program directors' committee report: topics related to controversial practices that should be taught in an allergy and immunology training program. J Allergy Clin Immunol. 1994;93:955–66.

SUGGESTED READINGS

Council on Scientific Affairs. In vivo diagnostic testing and immunology for allergy: report 1, part I of the Allergy Panel. JAMA. 1987;258:1363–7.

Council on Scientific Affairs. In vivo diagnostic testing and immunology for allergy: report 1, part II of the Allergy Panel. JAMA. 1987;258:1505–7.

Hamilton RG. Laboratory analyses in the diagnosis of human allergic disease. Methods. 1997;13:25–32.

Hamilton RG, Adkinson NF Jr. Measurement of total serum immunoglobulin E and allergen-specific immunoglobulin E antibody. In: Rose NR, de Macario EC, Fahey JL, Friedman H, Penn GM, eds. Manual of Clinical Laboratory Immunology. 4th ed. Washington, DC: American Society for Microbiology; 1992:689–701.

Lockey RF, Benedict LM, Turkeltaub PC, Bukantz SC. Fatalities from immunotherapy (IT) and skin testing (ST). J Allergy Clin Immunol. 1987;79:660–77.

Selner JC, Condemi J. Unproven diagnostic and therapeutic techniques for allergy. In: Middleton E Jr, Reed CE, Ellis EF, Adkinson NF Jr, Yunginger JW, eds. Allergy: Principles and Practice. 3rd ed. St. Louis: CV Mosby; 1988:1571–97.

Ten RM, Klein JS, Frigas E. Allergy skin testing. Mayo Clin Proc. 1995;70:783–4.

Chapter 2

Rhinitis

Phil Lieberman, MD

Impact and Epidemiology

Rhinitis may be the most common illness seen in the outpatient practice of medicine. Approximately 40 million people in the United States suffer from the allergic form of rhinitis, making it the most common IgE-mediated disease (1). Its economic impact is significant because the cost of therapy of allergic rhinitis in the United States is $1.23 billion annually. Rhinitis results in 824,000 missed school days, 811,000 missed work days, and 4,232,000 reduced-activity days (1). In addition, the chronic nonallergic form of rhinitis occurs with at least equal frequency in adults.

The mean age of onset of allergic rhinitis is between 8 and 11 years. The prevalence of the allergic form of rhinitis decreases with age; however, the mean onset of nonallergic rhinitis is much later in life, probably after 40 years of age. There is an equal incidence in men and women, and there are no known ethnic or racial differences in incidence.

The Nose as an Organ

The functions of the nose are shown in Box 2.1. These functions are carried out by the nasal turbinates. Turbinate swelling and shrinking is under the control of the autonomic nervous system. Sympathetic stimulation empties venous sinusoids within the turbinates, thus reducing their dimensions.

Box 2.1 Functions of the Nose

Breathing (conduit for air flow)
Air processing
  Humidification
  Warming
  Filtering
  Microbial defense
    Antibacterial
    Antiviral
Olfaction
Nasal reflection
Vocal resonation

Parasympathetic stimulation produces the opposite effect and also increases nasal secretions. Factors that exaggerate turbinate swelling and result in increased nasal congestion include lying flat, chilling the skin, and breathing cold air. On the other hand, aerobic exercise and warming the skin are natural nasal decongestants.

Diagnosis and Differential Diagnosis

The clinical expression of diseases of the nose is limited. The symptoms are congestion, postnasal drainage, rhinorrhea, sneezing, loss of olfaction, or any combination of these. The various forms of rhinitis are shown in Box 2.2. In the practice of internal medicine, the most commonly seen forms are allergic and chronic nonallergic rhinitis. The history is by far the most important tool used to establish the etiology of rhinitis. Essential features of the history are shown in Box 2.3. The key features distinguishing the two most common forms, allergic and chronic nonallergic rhinitis, are noted in Table 2.1.

The age of onset of allergic rhinitis is usually before 20 years, whereas chronic nonallergic rhinitis usually begins after 30 years. Allergic rhinitis may be seasonal or perennial. The most common seasons of exacerbation are spring and autumn during periods of pollination. Chronic nonallergic rhinitis is usually perennial but may also show exacerbations during periods of weather change, such as during late autumn and early spring. Most patients with seasonal allergic rhinitis show clear-cut exacerbations on exposure to aeroallergens, such as fresh-cut grass and animal dander. On the other hand, patients with chronic nonallergic rhinitis are characteristically made worse by

Box 2.2 Differential Diagnosis of Rhinitis

Allergic
>   *Seasonal*
>   *Perennial*

Chronic idiopathic nonallergic
>   *Nonallergic rhinitis with eosinophilia*
>   *Neurogenic (vasomotor)*

Mechanical–anatomic obstruction
>   *Polyps*
>   *Tumors*
>   *Granulomas*
>   *Sarcoid*
>   *Wegener's granulomatosis*
>   *Septal deviation*
>   *Septal perforation*
>   *Foreign bodies*

Drug-induced (rhinitis medicamentosa)
>   *Topical agents*
>   α-Adrenergic vasoconstrictors
>   Cocaine
>   Eye drops
>   *Oral agents*
>   Birth control pills
>   Antihypertensives
>   Phenothiazines

Acute cholinergic-induced
>   *Gustatory*
>   *Skier's–jogger's nose*

Endocrinologic
>   *Pregnancy*
>   *Hypothyroidism*
>   *Acromegaly*

Cerebrospinal leakage

Atrophic

Infectious

exposure to respiratory irritants, such as perfumes and cigarette smoke. Pruritus and paroxysms of sneezing are more commonly found in allergic rhinitis. In addition, patients with allergic rhinitis often manifest other symptoms of al-

Box 2.3   Important Elements of the History Useful To Establish the Cause of Rhinitis

Age of onset
Exacerbating factors
   Allergens
      Fresh-cut grass, animal dander, house dust, hay
   Irritants
      Cigarette smoke, odors, perfumes, detergents, soap powder
      Particulate dust
      Automobile exhaust fumes
   Weather conditions
      Weather fronts
      Humidity or temperature changes
      Damp, humid air
      Cold air
   Ingestants
      Alcohol
      Spicy foods
      Other
Nature of symptoms
   Sneezing
   Congestion
   Postnasal drainage
   Pruritus
   Anterior rhinorrhea
   Unilateral versus bilateral
Chronologic variations in symptoms
   Perennial without seasonal variation
   Perennial with seasonal variation
   Seasonal
      If seasonal or with seasonal variation, denote specific months
Environmental Exposures
   Workplace
   Home
   Pets
   Feathers
   Air-conditioning, heating
Hobbies/activities
Medications
   Oral
      Antihypertensives
      Birth control pills
      Tranquilizers
   Nasal sprays, eye drops
Family history of atopy
Other personal manifestations of atopy
Asthma
Allergic conjunctivitis
Atopic dermatitis

Table 2.1 Differential Diagnosis Between Allergic and Nonallergic Rhinitis

Manifestation	Allergic Rhinitis	Chronic Nonallergic Rhinitis
Age of onset	Usually before 20 y	Usually after 30 y
Seasonality	Usually with seasonal variation, spring and fall	Usually perennial but not infrequently worse during weather changes such as occur during fall and early spring
Exacerbating factors	Allergen exposure	Irritant exposure, weather conditions
Nature of symptoms		
Pruritus	Common	Rare
Congestion	Common	Common
Sneezing	Prominent	Usually not prominent but can be dominant in some cases
Postnasal drainage	Not prominent	Prominent
Other related manifestations (e.g., allergic, conjunctivitis, atopic dermatitis)	Often present	Absent
Family history	Usually present	Usually absent
Physical appearance	Variable, classically described as pale, boggy, swollen mucosa; may appear normal	Variable, erythematous
Allergy testing	Allergy skin tests always positive	Allergy skin tests negative or not clinically significant
Nasal eosinophilia	Usually present	Present 15%–20% of the time (nonallergic rhinitis with eosinophilia)

lergy, such as allergic conjunctivitis, atopic dermatitis, or allergic asthma. There is usually a family history of atopic disease in subjects with allergic rhinitis.

The physical examination can be deceiving. The classic description of a pale, boggy, cyanotic-appearing mucosa related to the presence of allergy is often absent. In fact, the nasal mucosa may appear normal in cases of allergic rhinitis. The appearance of the nasal mucosa in chronic nonallergic rhinitis is also highly variable. In fact, the value of physical examination of the nose is to rule out mechanical causes of rhinitis, such as nasal polyps, tumors, septal deviations, synechia, and septal perforations. In most instances, an adequate nasal examination can be accomplished using a strong light source and a nasal speculum. Fiberoptic rhinoscopy is ideal but need not be performed in every case.

Ancillary studies can be helpful. Nasal eosinophilia is usually present in allergic forms of the disease during exacerbations; however, 15% to 20% of patients with nonallergic rhinitis may also exhibit nasal eosinophilia. Patients with nonallergic rhinitis and eosinophilia are said to have nonallergic rhinitis with eosinophilia syndrome (NARES). The presence of eosinophilia is an important clinical point because it indicates the likelihood that corticosteroid therapy will be highly effective, regardless of whether the patient has allergic or nonallergic rhinitis.

The gold standard for the diagnosis of allergic rhinitis is the allergy skin test. In vitro testing can also be performed but is usually much more expensive and less sensitive.

Case 2.1

A 48-year-old woman presented with complaints of sneezing, itchy eyes, rhinorrhea, and nasal congestion dating back to childhood. She had not had adequate relief with over-the-counter antihistamines. The symptoms have been perennial but are worse during the months of May and September. She thought that she was worsened by exposure to fresh-cut grass. Her symptoms were also exacerbated to some extent by secondary cigarette smoke. The symptoms bothered her at all times during the day and occasionally awakened her from sleep at night. There was associated itching of the soft palate. The environmental history revealed two cats in the home.

The physical examination showed modestly swollen turbinates. No polyps were noted.

A nasal smear showed 75% eosinophilia (100 cells counted). Allergy skin tests performed by the prick method revealed positive reactions to grass pollen, weed pollen, and cats. (See Case 2.2 for discussions of diagnosis and treatment.)

Case 2.2

A 50-year-old man presented with a history of chronic nasal congestion and postnasal drainage dating back 6 years. Symptoms were perennial but showed seasonal exacerbations during changes of season. He thought that his worst symptoms occurred during the months of November, February, and March. He could "tell when a front was coming in" because he developed increased nasal congestion and often headaches located over the frontal and maxillary regions bilaterally when the weather changed. He had a poor response to antihistamine–decongestants. The symptoms were particularly bad at night. As soon as his "head hit the pillow," he developed significant congestion. Some degree of relief occurred when he jogged. The environmental history revealed that he has two cats and a dog at home.

The physical examination showed erythematous and swollen turbinates. There was posterior pharyngeal hyperplasia.

> ### Case 2.2 (continued)
>
> A nasal smear showed 30% eosinophilia (100 cells counted). Allergy skin tests were negative to an extensive battery of aeroallergens. Sinus radiographs were normal.
>
> This case and Case 2.1 illustrate two of the most common forms of chronic rhinitis. The first case is a woman with perennial allergic rhinitis, and the second is a man with chronic nonallergic rhinitis. The gold standard to distinguish between these two entities is the allergy skin test; however, clues in the history are very important. In Case 2.1, the presence of itching that worsens on exposure to aeroallergens and spring and autumn exacerbations consistent with the pollen seasons point to an allergic etiology. In Case 2.2, the failure of symptoms to be exacerbated by allergens and the fact that the seasonal increases in symptoms were more consistent with weather changes than with pollen seasons indicate a diagnosis of nonallergic rhinitis.
>
> Of importance is the presence of eosinophilia. Eosinophils are not, per se, a sign of allergy. Nasal eosinophilia can occur in approximately 25% of patients with nonallergic rhinitis. This condition, known as NARES, mimics allergic disease. The significance of eosinophils is that corticosteroid treatment usually elicits a good response.
>
> In Case 2.1, an obvious factor in therapy would be to remove the pets from the home. This would, of course, not be indicated in Case 2.2. The medication regimen for each, however, would be very similar: a short burst of oral corticosteroids, topical nasal corticosteroids administered on a regular basis, and antihistamine–decongestants on an as-needed basis.

Although the most common forms of rhinitis encountered in the practice of internal medicine are allergic and nonallergic, it is important to consider other possibilities in each case. Nasal obstruction produced by mechanical or anatomic lesions is easily missed without an adequate physical examination. Obstructive lesions consist of nasal polyps, tumors, granulomas, septal deviation, and foreign bodies. In addition, turbinate swelling that causes obstructive symptoms can be seen in sarcoidosis and Wegener's granulomatosis. Also of note is that some people with septal perforation complain of nasal obstruction due to disturbances of intranasal air flow. Such disturbances are perceived as obstruction even though nasal patency is normal. Clues to the presence of mechanical obstruction are the absence of other symptoms of rhinitis, such as sneezing, rhinorrhea, and itching.

Several differential diagnostic features can be used to distinguish nasal polyps from tumors. Polyps are usually bilateral and tumors are usually unilateral. Although both can be associated with nasal bleeding, as a rule tumors bleed far more readily and copiously than do polyps. Polyps also have a different appearance on physical examination; they usually appear mucoid and smooth, whereas tumors often appear granulomatous and erythematous. Polyps are sessile and easily and painlessly manipulated, whereas tumors are usually more fixed and painful if manipulated. Both are associated with sinusitis.

Rhinitis medicamentosa can be due to both topical and oral agents. The most frequent cause is the overuse of topical vasoconstrictor agents that can be purchased over the counter. Eye drops gain access to the nose through the nasal lacrimal ducts and can also produce rhinitis medicamentosa on rare occasions. Numerous oral agents (e.g., birth control pills, antihypertensives, and phenothiazines) can cause drug-induced rhinitis. Nasal congestion is the major complaint related to the overuse of topical nose drops.

Cholinergic rhinitis is characterized by the sudden onset of profuse rhinorrhea and is due to stimulation of the cholinergic nervous system. Typical cases occur when eating, especially spicy food (gustatory rhinitis), and on exposure to cold air, such as while jogging in the winter or skiing ("skier's–jogger's nose"). Such patients suffer from a copious watery rhinorrhea. The symptoms begin almost simultaneously with exposure to the appropriate stimulus.

Case 2.3

A 68-year-old man presented with a history of profuse rhinorrhea. The symptoms were perennial, not related to exposure to aeroallergens, but exacerbated by cold air and by eating. In fact, the rhinorrhea that occurred during eating has made him reluctant to socialize during meals. The rhinorrhea was clear and had the appearance of water. There was no associated sneezing or nasal congestion.

The ear, nose, and throat examination was without abnormality, and sinus radiographs were normal.

A nasal eosinophil smear failed to reveal eosinophils, and allergy skin tests were negative.

This patient illustrates a case of cholinergic rhinorrhea due to hyperactive cholinergic reflexes usually stimulated by cold air exposure or by eating (especially spicy food).

This condition responds well to a topical anticholinergic agent (ipratropium bromide [Atrovent]). Two squirts in each nostril of the 0.06% or 0.03% preparations taken approximately an hour before eating or exposure to cold air are highly effective. In this case, the patient responded well to this therapy.

There are a number of forms of endocrinologic rhinitis. Rhinitis of pregnancy is perhaps the most common. The vascular receptors are sensitive to estrogen and progesterone. In some women, the sensitivity to these agents (which produce vasodilatation) seems to be excessive. This sensitivity coupled with an increase in blood volume produces nasal congestion, which progresses in severity during pregnancy and subsides at parturition. Hypothyroidism can also be associated with turbinate congestion. The turbinates are very sensitive to growth hormone and, therefore, hypertrophy can occur in subjects with acromegaly. Endocrinologic rhinitis usually can be distinguished from allergic rhinitis by the absence of sneezing, itching, and rhinorrhea.

Atrophic rhinitis usually occurs in the elderly but can occur at any age. In this condition, there is a decreased mucus flow, resulting in drying of the nasal mucosa. There is often secondary bacterial infection.

Cerebral spinal fluid (CSF) leakage is rare and therefore requires a high index of suspicion to establish the diagnosis. In most instances, it is associated with head trauma or surgery, but it should be noted that CSF leakage can occur without any history of head trauma or other central nervous system pathology. In this disorder, patients complain of a profuse watery rhinorrhea that can be unilateral or bilateral. There usually is no clear-cut precipitating or exacerbating factor; however, upon "straining down" or "leaning forward" there is usually an increase in liquid flow. Many times, such patients can collect fluid in a beaker by simply leaning forward. A simple diagnostic test is the "glucose dipstick." Normal nasal secretions do not contain glucose, whereas those associated with CSF rhinorrhea will contain levels one third that of blood.

Pathogenesis of Allergic Rhinitis

Allergic rhinitis is a prototype of IgE mediated diseases. Within minutes of allergen challenge, mast cells within the nasal mucosa degranulate. Mediators, such as histamine and products of arachidonic acid, are released and symptoms occur almost instantaneously. In addition, chemotactic factors are released, and there is up-regulation of adhesion molecules on vascular endothelium. These molecules, such as VCAM-1 and ICAM-1, serve as binding anchors for circulating cells called to the site by the chemotactic agents; thus, by 3 hours after allergen challenge, there is a rich infiltration of cells into the nasal mucosa and submucosa. The predominant cell is the eosinophil, but neutrophils and basophils also appear. The infiltration of these cells is characterized by a recrudescence of nasal symptoms.

The allergic reaction appears to occur in two phases. Acute symptoms (the early phase) begin within minutes of exposure to allergen and usually abate within an hour. This early-phase reaction is caused by rapidly acting mediators released by mast cells. A few hours later, symptoms recur due to the influx of the cells noted above. This later recrudescence in symptoms is known as the *late-phase reaction.*

Continued exposure to allergen will lead to more chronic inflammatory changes within the nasal mucosa. From this, a state of hyperirritability will occur. The patient then becomes more sensitive not only to allergen challenge but also to irritant challenge. Chronic allergen exposure, therefore, produces a far more profound effect than the immediate onset of nasal symptoms.

The pathogenesis of chronic nonallergic rhinitis is unclear. This disorder is actually not one illness but rather a diagnosis of exclusion; that is, chronic symptoms that cannot be accounted for by other reasons are designated as due to chronic nonallergic rhinitis. The clinical manifestations of this condition are therefore not as uniform as those of allergic rhinitis.

Therapy

The pharmacopeia for therapy of rhinitis has been greatly enriched over the past decade. The drugs available for therapy now include H_1 antihistamines, decongestants, cromolyn sodium, anticholinergics, and corticosteroids. Nonpharmacologic measures, such as environmental control and allergen immunotherapy, are effective measures as well.

Pharmacologic Therapy

Antihistamines

All H_1 antihistamines are competitive antagonists of histamine and have been conveniently classified into first- and second-generation families. Some of the commonly used first-generation antihistamines are diphenhydramine, chlorpheniramine, hydroxyzine, and azatadine.

All first-generation antihistamines cause drowsiness to some extent. In addition, they have varying anticholinergic activities. These two characteristics have limited their usefulness in many instances. Second-generation antihistamines (Table 2.2) do not cause drowsiness nor do they have a markedly attenuated potential to do so.

All antihistamines are rapidly absorbed from the gastrointestinal tract. With the exception of two second-generation antihistamines (cetirizine and fexofenadine), all are metabolized via the cytochrome P_{450} system; therefore, hepatic dysfunction or drugs that interfere with cytochrome P_{450} activity can prolong the half-life of these drugs. This is of clinical importance with astemizole, because interference with its metabolism results in the accumulation of agents that have cardiotoxicity and the potential of producing ventricular arrhythmias (most notably torsades de pointes). The production of arrhythmias by these drugs is thought to be due to prolongation of the QT interval produced by interference with the delayed potassium rectifier channel (2).

Antihistamines are most effective for sneezing, pruritus, and rhinorrhea. They exert little effect on nasal congestion; therefore, as a rule, they are more effective in acute, seasonal allergic rhinitis than in the chronic perennial form in which congestion is usually more prominent. They are also, as a rule, more effective in allergic than in chronic nonallergic rhinitis.

As noted, the most important side effect of first-generation antihistamines is drowsiness. Approximately one third of patients taking first-generation drugs complain of this side effect; however, some patients who do not actually detect drowsiness still exhibit reduced reaction time, inability to concentrate, and the blunting of other cognitive functions. This is of importance because it means that patients may be at risk when operating machinery, driving, and so forth, even though they do not notice impairment. Drowsiness itself can be overcome by conscious effort, but impairment of function without drowsiness persists until the effect of the drug abates (3).

First-generation antihistamines also can cause side effects via their antimuscarinic activity. These include urinary retention and dysuria, blurring of vision, dry mouth, and constipation.

As noted, second-generation antihistamines do not cause drowsiness. In addition, they do not have anticholinergic activity. At the present time, four second-generation drugs are available for use. These are astemizole (Hismanal), fexofenadine (Allegra), loratadine (Claritin), and cetirizine (Zyrtec). As noted, astemizole has been associated with ventricular arrhythmias. For this reason, its use has declined. Loratadine, fexofenadine, and cetirizine have not been associated with prolongation of the QT interval or ventricular arrhythmias. These drugs have specific characteristics (*see* Table 2.2), which give them distinct clinical profiles. For example, in contrast to loratadine and astemizole, the liver is not the major source of metabolism of cetirizine and fexofenadine. The

Table 2.2 Characteristics of Second-Generation Antihistamines

Drug Name	Dosage	Sedative Potential	Associated with Ventricular Arrhythmia?	Major Route of Metabolism/Secretion	Available with Decongestant?	Useful as Rapid Onset "prn" Drugs?
Astemizole (Hismanal)	10 mg qd	None	Yes	Liver	No	No
Loratadine (Claritin)	10 mg qd	None	No	Liver	Yes (pseudo-ephedrine; qd or bid dosage)	Yes
Cetirizine (Zyrtec)	10 mg qd	Reduced but present	No	Kidney	No	Yes
Fexofenadine (Allegra)	60 mg bid	None	No	Mainly unmetabolized; 80% found in feces	Yes (pseudo-ephedrine; qd or bid dosage)	Yes

majority of both of these drugs is excreted in the urine; thus, their dose should be reduced in patients with renal insufficiency. Astemizole requires some degree of tissue accumulation before it reaches peak effect. It is therefore not suitable for "prn" use because its maximum onset of activity is usually delayed until three doses have been administered. All of these drugs (except cetirizine) have been rated as nonsedating antihistamines by the Federal Drug Administration. Cetirizine has a low sedating potential.

Traditionally, antihistamines have been administered orally. Recently, a topically administered antihistamine (azelastine via nose spray) was introduced. Azelastine has an indication for use in seasonal allergic rhinitis. It is administered in a dose of two squirts in each nostril twice per day. It has an onset of action within 1 hour, its activity shows statistical significance over placebo within 2 to 3 hours, and its duration of activity is 12 hours. It does not produce any significant electrocardiographic abnormalities, and although it is hepatically metabolized, it does not interact with ketoconazole, erythromycin, theophylline, cimetidine, or ranitidine. However, in contrast to the second-generation antihistamines noted above, azelastine does have some sedative potential and anticholinergic activity.

Decongestants

All nasal decongestants are α-adrenergic drugs. They act by contracting the vascular sphincters located proximal to the venous plexuses of the turbinates. They are effective only for turbinate swelling and exert little effect on other manifestations of rhinitis. They are more effective topically than orally; however, topical use can result in rhinitis medicamentosa and therefore should be limited to 1 week. Topically, their onset of action is within minutes; orally, it is within approximately 1 hour. Topical decongestants have a role in the therapy of sinusitis, upper respiratory tract infections, and the prevention of barotrauma and otitis related to air travel. Oral decongestants have a role in the therapy of chronic rhinitis.

The number of decongestants is limited (Box 2.4). There is no clear-cut drug of choice. The long-acting topical agents oxymetazoline and xylometazoline are probably superior to shorter-acting drugs if for no other reason than convenience.

Oral decongestants usually can be administered without significant side effects. The most common side effects are nervousness, insomnia, and difficulty with urination (especially in patients with prostatism). Other side effects are infrequent. Although there is a well-known admonition not to prescribe these drugs to patients with hypertension, they actually appear to be safe in subjects with stable hypertension (4). Because antihistamines have little effect on congestion and decongestants have little effect on other symptoms of rhinitis, these two drugs are commonly employed as combination agents.

Box 2.4 Decongestants

Oral
    Pseudoephedrine
    Phenylpropanolamine
    Phenylephrine
Topical long-acting (8–12 h)
    Oxymetazoline
    Xylometazoline
Topical short-acting (3–8 h)
    Tetrahydrozoline
    Naphazoline
    Phenylephrine

Anticholinergics

Anticholinergic agents are most useful for anterior watery rhinorrhea. They are the drugs of choice for treatment of gustatory rhinitis and skier's–jogger's nose. They are also useful in alleviating anterior rhinorrhea associated with viral infections of the upper respiratory tract.

Ipratropium bromide is a topical anticholinergic agent that is available in an aqueous solution. It can be obtained in both a 0.03% and 0.06% solution. Ipratropium bromide is an analog of atropine and has an advantage over atropine because it does not cross the blood–brain barrier or slow mucociliary clearance; thus, it can be administered in most patients totally without side effect.

The 0.03% solution is indicated for the therapy of chronic rhinitis, and the 0.06% solution is useful for anterior rhinorrhea associated with the common cold. Both drugs can be helpful in preventing symptoms due to gustatory rhinitis or skier's–jogger's nose. The most common side effect is nasal irritation.

Anticholinergic agents available as belladonna alkaloids are also found in some antihistamine–decongestant combination drugs. In oral forms, these drugs are also highly effective for rhinorrhea; however, they can cause side effects of drowsiness, dry mouth, and difficulty urinating. Nonetheless, they may be highly useful administered at night when drowsiness is desirable.

Cromolyn Sodium

Cromolyn sodium is useful for seasonal allergic rhinitis and in preventing symptoms due to isolated allergen exposure, and it is now available over the counter. For seasonal allergic rhinitis, cromolyn sodium is usually started before the onset of symptoms and continued for an entire allergy season. To prevent symptoms due to isolated allergen exposure (e.g., when mowing the lawn), the drug is administered immediately before exposure. Cromolyn sodium has a duration of activity of approximately 4 to 6 hours. It is not as effective as topical corticosteroids and requires a more inconvenient dosing schedule.

Corticosteroids

Corticosteroids are the most effective drugs for the therapy of both allergic and nonallergic rhinitis; oral therapy is usually more effective than topical therapy. A 10-day tapering course of prednisone beginning at 50 mg per day is almost universally effective in controlling all symptoms of rhinitis. Oral corticosteroid therapy is recommended before the initiation of topical therapy in patients with active symptoms. Pretreatment with oral corticosteroids can speed the onset of relief and prevent exacerbations of symptoms when topical therapy is applied to an inflamed nasal mucosa. Six drugs are available for topical use (Table 2.3). All of these drugs have a high topical-to-systemic ratio of activity and cause no detectable systemic effect in recommended doses. In addition, topical side effects are minimal, even after long-term use. Nasal irritation is probably the most common side effect. Nasal bleeding, especially when blowing the nose, also can occur with significant frequency. Nasal septal perforation is a rare complication, but patients should be monitored for the occurrence of this side effect. It is thought that the side effect occurs more frequently if the spray is directed to the nasal septum; therefore, patients should be instructed to point the spray toward the ear of the side being treated to avoid contact with the septum. Although rare cases of elevation of intraocular pressure have been reported, the risk of glaucoma is minimal, as is the incidence of cataracts.

It is clear that these drugs are safe for use during seasonal allergic rhinitis; however, it is unclear exactly how long they can be used without risk of side effects. Nonetheless, nasal biopsy specimens obtained from patients using beclomethasone continually for several years have shown no significant mucosal atrophy (5).

There is no clear-cut drug of choice among topically available corticosteroids. Some of the preparations are scented (fluticasone and beclomethasone aqueous preparations) and come in either aqueous or aerosol preparations, but these options are related to patient preference and not to efficacy or incidence of side effects.

Format for Pharmacologic Therapy

With the knowledge of the pharmacology and characteristics of each therapeutic agent, a suggested format for therapy of rhinitis can be constructed. The agents employed should vary according to the severity of the symptoms and the patient's ability to tolerate individual drugs. For mild symptoms, an antihistamine or an antihistamine–decongestant alone might be sufficient. For symptoms of rhinorrhea, sneezing, and itching, the antihistamine alone would be sufficient. If congestion is the sole symptom, then a decongestant alone is appropriate. For combinations of sneezing, rhinorrhea, itching, and congestion, a combination drug is indicated. Because of cost considerations, sedating antihistamines may be considered, especially for bedtime use. Many potentially sedating agents are available over the counter as combination antihistamine–decongestants. Examples of these are Dimetapp (brompheniramine/phenylpropanolamine) and Tavist-D (clemastine/phenylpropanolamine). In addition, there is a wide variety of agents containing combinations of chlorpheniramine with either phenylpropanolamine or pseudoephedrine; however, if sedation occurs or there is concern over impairment of performance without overt sedation, then, of course, a

Table 2.3 Topical Corticosteroid Preparations Used To Treat Rhinitis

Drug	Brand Name	Type of Delivery	Dosage	Sprays per Container
Beclomethasone	Beconase or Vancenase	Fluorocarbon aerosol	1 spray in each nostril bid to qid (1 spray = 42 mg)	200
	Beconase AQ or Vancenase AQ	Liquid spray	1–2 sprays each nostril bid (1 spray = 42 mg)	200
	Vancenase AQDS	Liquid spray	1–2 sprays each nostril qd (1 spray = 84 mg)	120
Triamcinolone	Nasacort	Fluorocarbon aerosol	1–2 sprays each nostril qd to bid (1 spray = 55 mg)	100
	Nasacort AQ	Liquid spray	1–2 sprays each nostril qd (1 spray = 55 mg)	120
Flunisolide	Nasarel	Liquid spray	1–2 sprays each nostril bid (1 spray = 25 mg)	200
Budesonide	Rhinocort	Fluorocarbon aerosol	4 sprays each nostril qd (1 spray =32 mg)	200
Fluticasone	Flonase	Liquid spray	1–2 sprays each nostril qd (1 spray =50 mg)	120
Mometasone	Nasonex	Liquid spray	2 sprays each nostril qd (1 spray =50 mg)	240

nonsedating antihistamine is preferable. If an antihistamine alone is indicated, there are several choices, including loratadine (Claritin), fexofenadine (Allegra), and cetirizine (Zyrtec), which is a low-sedating alternative. At the time of publication, two of these are available with a decongestant: loratadine (Claritin-D) and fexofenadine (Allegra-D). One possible compromise between cost and potential side effects is to prescribe a sedating antihistamine or antihistamine–decongestant at night along with a 12-hour nonsedating preparation in the morning.

When symptoms are not adequately controlled by antihistamine–decongestants, intranasal steroids are recommended. These are given on a regular basis, and the antihistamine–decongestant combinations are used as a supplement as needed. When symptoms are severe and interfere with normal activities and sleep (particularly in the midst of a pollen season), oral corticosteroids can be added to the regimen. A brief course of steroids beginning with 40 mg daily and tapering to discontinuation over 5 to 7 days is highly effective in achieving control during such times. The nasal corticosteroid should be continued during the course of oral corticosteroid treatment.

Pharmacologic Therapy of Specific Forms of Rhinitis

Mild seasonal allergic rhinitis or perennial allergic rhinitis usually can be controlled with antihistamines or antihistamine–decongestant combinations. Symptoms not responding to these agents require topical corticosteroids or topical cromolyn sodium. In more severe forms, a combination of a topical corticosteroid and ipratropium bromide may be helpful. The effect of these two drugs administered together has been shown to be superior to either administered alone.

Rhinitis medicamentosa should be treated with a taper of oral corticosteroids over a week to 10 days. On the third day of administration, a topical corticosteroid is added to the regimen. The topical corticosteroid is used for a minimum of 1 month. The drug producing the rhinitis medicamentosa should be discontinued within 1 week of the initiation of oral corticosteroids. Oral decongestants are employed as needed.

Gustatory rhinitis and skier's–jogger's nose respond to the inhalation of ipratropium bromide before exposure (eating or exercising in the cold). Either the 0.03% or 0.06% preparation can be used. The drug should be administered approximately 1 hour before eating or exercising.

Rhinitis of pregnancy is a particularly difficult problem because of the admonition not to use drugs during pregnancy. In addition, symptoms are often somewhat resistant to medication (with the exception of topical corticosteroids, which are generally considered to be safe in pregnancy). The decision to initiate pharmacologic therapy should be taken in conjunction with the obstetrician. The condition usually worsens as the pregnancy proceeds.

Nonpharmacologic Therapy

Patients with allergic rhinitis should take measures to control environmental exposure. For example, if the patient is allergic to animals, ideally he or she should not have an indoor pet. Often the removal of a pet from the home can alleviate symptoms entirely. Other exposures, such as mowing the lawn, dusting the home, and so forth, should be avoided if the patient demonstrates symptoms during these activities. Air-conditioning during pollen season is also very helpful.

Allergen immunotherapy is an effective tool used to alleviate symptoms of allergic rhinitis, especially in its seasonal form, and is discussed in Chapter 10. Saline nose sprays, humidification, and other measures may be helpful in individual patients.

Complications of Rhinitis

Perhaps the most important complication of rhinitis (Box 2.5) is not relevant to the field of internal medicine, but it is extremely important in pediatrics. A number of prominent abnormalities in facial development occur in children with severe, perennial rhinitis. These occur due to chronic mouth breathing; therefore, it is essential to vigorously treat children and adolescents who have severe rhinitis.

Otitis media and sinusitis occur whenever there is obstruction of the eustachian tube, sinus ostia, or both. Rhinitis is one of the most common causes of obstruction and, therefore, clearly predisposes to these two disorders. Correction of nasal obstruction is essential in the therapy of both.

A number of studies suggest that uncontrolled rhinitis aggravates bronchoconstriction. The exact reasons why rhinitis adversely affects asthma are

---

Box 2.5 Complications of Rhinitis

Disturbances of facial growth and development
    Increased length of face
    Retrognathic maxilla and mandible
    Cross-bite
    High, arched palate
Otitis media
Sinusitis
Disturbance of taste and smell
Sleep interruption and sleep apnea
Activation of nasal–bronchial reflexes

unclear but are believed to be related to nasal bronchial reflexes and failure to condition the air before it enters the lung. Control of rhinitis, therefore, is necessary for the optimal control of asthma.

Although rhinitis rarely causes sleep apnea, it certainly can aggravate this condition; apneic episodes clearly increase in frequency when nasal obstruction is present. The correction of rhinitis is essential for optimal control of sleep apnea.

REFERENCES

1. **Malone DC, Lawson KA, Smith DH, et al.** A cost of illness study of allergic rhinitis in the United States. J Allergy Clin Immunol. 1997;99:22–7.
2. **Kemp JP.** Antihistamines: Is there anything safe to prescribe? Ann Allergy. 1992; 69:276–80.
3. **Druce H.** Impairment of function by antihistamines. Ann Allergy. 1990;64:403–5.
4. **Kroenke K, Omori D, Simmons J, Wood D, Meier N.** The safety of phenyl-propanolamine in patients with stable hypertension. Ann Int Med. 1989; 3:1043–4.
5. **Mygand N, Sorensen H, Peterson CB.** The nasal mucosa during long-term treatment with beclomethasone dipropionate aerosol: a light and scanning electron microscopic study of nasal polyps. Acta Otolaryngol. 1978;85:437–43.

SUGGESTED READING

Hogan MB, Grammar LC, Patterson R. Rhinitis [Review]. Ann Allergy. 1994;72:293–300.

Kobayashi RH, Kiechel F, Kobayashi ALD, Mellion MB. Topical nasal sprays: treatment of allergic rhinitis. Am Fam Physician. 1994;50:151–7.

Lieberman P. Rhinitis. In: Lieberman P and Anderson J, eds. Allergic Diseases: Diagnosis and Treatment. Totowa, NJ: Humana Press, Inc.; 1997:323–30.

Lund VJ. Seasonal allergic rhinitis: a review of current therapy. Allergy. 1996;51(Suppl 28):5–7.

Meltzer EO. The prevalence and medical and economic impact of allergic rhinitis in the United States. J Allergy Clin Immunol. 1997;99(Suppl):S805–28.

Chapter 3

Sinusitis

Raymond G. Slavin, MD

Prevalence and Impact on Quality of Life

Sinusitis accounts for 11.6 million physician office visits per year and is the fifth leading cause for antibiotic usage. It is the most frequently reported chronic disease in the United States, affecting 14.7% of the population.

In a 36-item health survey used to determine general health assessment, patients with sinusitis showed significant decrease in bodily pain, general health, vitality, and social functioning. Sinusitis patients scored lower in bodily pain and social functioning than patients with chronic obstructive pulmonary disease, congestive heart failure, angina, and back pain.

It has been suggested that the term *rhinosinusitis* may be more accurate than *sinusitis* because 1) rhinitis typically precedes sinusitis, 2) sinusitis without rhinitis is rare, 3) the mucosa of the nose and sinuses are contiguous, and 4) symptoms of nasal obstruction and discharge are prominent in sinusitis (1).

How the Sinuses Become Infected

Patency of the ostia is the most important factor in the development of sinusitis. If the ostia—the small openings in the lateral wall of the nose through which the sinuses drain—are obstructed, two things happen that predispose to infection: 1) secretions produced by the sinus mucosa accumulate and stagnate; and

2) gas exchange is impaired, resulting in a decrease in sinus P_{O_2} and an increase in sinus P_{CO_2}. The mucociliary apparatus is also important in the protection against infection. Micro-organisms and foreign particles that escape the filtering process in the nose are trapped in the mucus of the sinuses and are removed through the ostia by constant movement of the mucous blanket and propelled by the underlying cilia. When this self-cleansing mechanism is impaired, bacterial infection occurs. Mucus accumulates, stagnates, and becomes infected by relatively harmless pyogenic bacteria normally found in the nose.

Mucociliary activity of the sinuses is particularly important because spontaneous drainage of the maxillary sinuses by gravity is nearly impossible for two reasons. Firstly, the maxillary ostium is located not in the inferior portion of the maxillary antrum (where gravity would favor drainage) but rather in the superior portion. Ciliary action, therefore, must move secretions up and out against the force of gravity. Secondly, the drainage area of the maxillary and ethmoid sinuses is a circuitous channel 6 to 8 mm long that connects the maxillary and ethmoid antra to the middle meatus. This is called the *ostiomeatal complex*, and its length and tortuous nature afford ample opportunity for obstruction.

Conditions That Predispose to Sinusitis

Understanding the pathophysiology of sinusitis enables physicians to determine logically the predisposing conditions (Box 3.1). The leading systemic condition that predisposes to sinusitis is immune deficiency. Patients with hy-

---

Box 3.1 Conditions Predisposing to Sinusitis

Systemic
    Immune deficiency
    Cystic fibrosis
    Dysmotile cilia syndrome
Local
    Viral upper respiratory infections
    Allergic rhinitis
    Deviated nasal septum
    Nasal polyps
    Foreign bodies
    Swimming and diving
    Smoking

pogammaglobulenemia have a high incidence of sinusitis; thus, it is apparent that immunoglobulins play an important role in defense against sinusitis. The incidence of sinusitis in AIDS patients may be as high as 68%. The organisms causing bacterial sinusitis in HIV-infected patients are similar to those reported in the general population, but AIDS patients with CD4 cell counts of less than 150 are susceptible to opportunistic organisms, such as cytomegalovirus, *Pseudomonas*, and fungi (2).

As important as the systemic conditions are, local factors are far more common. Sinusitis most commonly follows a viral upper respiratory infection. The acute rhinitis results in an edematous obstruction of the sinus ostium, negative pressure in the sinuses, and a decrease in paranasal sinus ciliary action. With the subsequent accumulation of mucus in the sinuses, the stage is set for secondary bacterial infection and the conversion of mucus to mucopus. The negative pressure in the sinuses favors aspiration of bacteria-laden material from the nose. Mucopus further impairs ciliary action and increases the swelling around the ostia when it discharges into the nose, thus creating a vicious cycle.

The association of allergy with sinusitis has not been fully elucidated, although a number of studies have suggested a specific relationship. An increased incidence of sinusitis has been found in children referred to an allergist–immunologist for evaluation of rhinitis. A large proportion of these children were proven to be atopic, supporting a connection between allergic rhinitis and sinus disease.

Microbiology

Knowledge of the true microbiotic picture in sinusitis has come from aseptic aspirates obtained by direct antral puncture or direct sampling during surgery. Cultures from both adults and children with acute sinusitis grow predominantly aerobic organisms, with *Streptococcus pneumoniae*, *Haemophilus influenzae*, and *Moraxella* (formerly *Branhamella*) *catarrhalis* being the most prevalent.

The role of microbial infection in chronic sinus disease is not clear. Generally, anaerobic organisms were thought to play the major pathogenic role in chronic sinusitis, but recent studies of patients scheduled for surgery revealed that aerobes were isolated in 76.3% of cases and anaerobes in only 7.6%. A hypothesis has been offered that bacterial infection has a minor role, if any, in chronic sinusitis in many patients.

Fungal infection of the paranasal sinuses may occur in both immunocompromised and immunocompetent individuals. *Aspergillus fumigatus* is the most common fungus found in both groups. *Mucor* sinusitis is particularly common in diabetic patients.

Case 3.1

A 36-year-old woman complained of a 3-month history of nasal congestion, post-nasal drainage, and sore throat. She was not able to describe her postnasal drainage because she swallowed it. Careful questioning revealed that her husband had commented on her strong breath.

Physical examination revealed swollen, reddened nasal turbinates, with purulent material in the nose and the pharynx.

Antibiotic therapy resulted in resolution of symptoms.

Diagnosis

History and Physical Examination

The most important clinical clue to the diagnosis of acute sinusitis is the failure of symptoms to resolve after a typical cold. The patient will note that nasal discharge that had previously been clear becomes yellow or green. Fever persists, chills may develop, and pain more severe on bending or straining is often felt in the cheek. On physical examination, thick, purulent green or deep-yellow secretions are seen most often in the middle meatus, which is the draining site of the maxillary sinus.

If mucopus is not evacuated, then acute sinusitis may enter a subacute or chronic phase. Here, the diagnostic index of suspicion of the physician must be high, for the typical clinical presentation of chronic sinusitis is subtle. The patient generally presents with nasal stuffiness, purulent postnasal drainage, sore throat, hyposmia, fetid breath, and malaise. On physical examination, an edematous and hyperemic nasal mucosa is generally bathed in mucopus. Nasal endoscopy may be useful for visualizing the middle meatus and the flow of infected mucus.

Nasal Smear and Culture

Microscopic examination of nasal secretions may be of great diagnostic value. In instances of bacterial sinusitis, one sees sheets of polymorphonuclear neutrophils and bacteria. This is unlike viral upper respiratory infections (in which polymorphonuclear neutrophils are scant) or allergic rhinitis (in which a high percentage of eosinophils may be seen). Nasal culture does not give an adequate picture of the organisms responsible for sinusitis. The true microbiologic picture of sinusitis can be obtained only by direct antral puncture.

Imaging Techniques

Two imaging modalities are used for the diagnosis of sinusitis: plain films and computed tomography (CT) scanning. Plain radiographs of the sinuses in adults have been shown to correlate with positive bacterial cultures when there is mucosal thickening of greater than 8 mm, an air–fluid level, or opacification. Conventional radiographs have the disadvantage of not delineating the status of individual ethmoid air cells or the ostiomeatal complex, nor can they accurately show the extent of inflammatory disease in affected patients. In short, many significant instances of sinusitis, particularly of the ethmoid sinuses, are missed on plain films (3). For these reasons, CT is the radiographic modality of choice to examine the paranasal sinuses (Fig. 3.1). Coronal CT scans demonstrate the ostiomeatal complex and may detect subtle disease not shown on plain radiographs. A limited four-slice coronal CT scan of the sinuses has been shown to provide much more information than plain films and at a much reduced radiation dose and cost than full CT. Positive CT scans of the sinuses are not specific for bacterial or fungal infections, because patients with naturally acquired common colds may demonstrate sinus abnormalities (4).

It must be emphasized that in the vast majority of cases, careful history and physical examination will suffice to make the diagnosis of sinusitis and institute appropriate therapy. Box 3.2 shows instances in which one might want to order a sinus CT examination.

Other Diagnostic Techniques

Transillumination in a carefully controlled study has been shown to be of limited use in the diagnosis of sinusitis. Ultrasound, although useful in detecting fluid in maxillary sinuses, has been shown to result in a high degree of false-positive and false-negative results. These techniques, therefore, cannot be recommended.

Medical Treatment

Medical therapy of acute sinusitis includes steam and saline instillation into the nose, topical or oral decongestants, mucus thinners, topical or systemic corticosteroids, and control of infection with antibiotics.

Topical decongestants may be useful in promoting sinus drainage, but they should be used for only 3 to 4 days to avoid the vasodilating rebound phenomenon that results in rhinitis medicamentosa.

In some cases of hyperplastic rhinosinusitis, with or without nasal polyps, systemic corticosteroids may be administered over a short period of time.

The antibiotics of choice for treatment of acute sinusitis are ampicillin and amoxicillin. The organisms previously mentioned as causing acute sinusitis are sensitive to these drugs, and there is good evidence that adequate mucosal

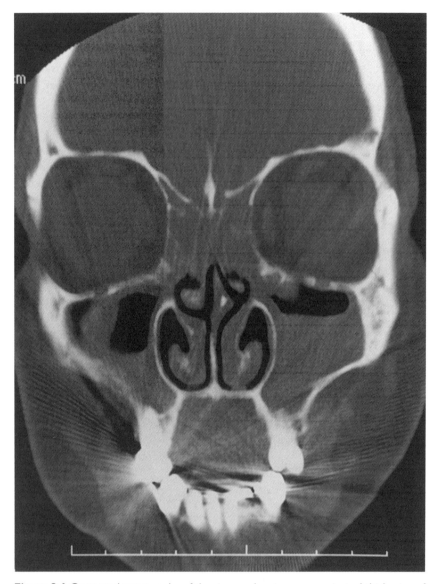

Figure 3.1 Computed tomography of the sinuses showing mucoperiosteal thickening of the maxillary sinuses, bilateral air–fluid levels, and opacification of the ethmoid sinuses.

and sinus fluid levels of these antibiotics are obtained. In the case of penicillin sensitivity, trimethoprim with sulfamethoxazole is an adequate alternative. Treatment of acute sinusitis should be 10 to 14 days in duration.

β-Lactamase–producing organisms have been recognized increasingly as a cause of sinusitis in both children and adults. Clavulanic acid, an inhibitor of

---

Box 3.2   When To Order a Computed Tomography Scan of the Sinuses

---

Failure to respond to therapy

Negative radiographs despite persistent signs and symptoms

Evaluation of anatomic abnormalities

Confirming improvement after prolonged course of antibiotics in chronic
    sinusitis

Localizing disease for possible surgery

Evaluate for complications

---

the β-lactamases, has been introduced in combination with amoxicillin for treatment of β-lactamase–producing organisms. Other antibiotics found to be useful in treating sinusitis are cefuroxime axetil, loracarbef, clarithromycin, and azithromycin. Chronic sinusitis may have to be treated for 3 to 4 weeks or longer.

Surgical Treatment

Persistent or recurrent episodes of sinusitis after appropriate medical therapy may indicate an anatomic problem that mandates surgical consideration. A wide spectrum of surgical procedures are available for treating medically resistant sinusitis, but functional endoscopic sinus surgery (FESS) has emerged as the technique of choice in most instances. The usefulness of the technique is predicated on the evidence that the middle meatus–anterior ethmoid complex (ostiomeatal unit) is heavily involved in the pathogenesis of sinusitis. The advantages of FESS are minimal trauma to normal nasal and sinus structures and conservative removal of infected tissue; thus, a return to the natural physiology and mucociliary clearance and function of the sinuses is made possible.

Complications

Extension of Infection

The most commonly seen extensions of infections are orbital and include cellulitis, abscess, and cavernous sinus thrombosis. Intracranial extension of infection may result in epidural or subdural abscess. Mucocele formation and osteomyelitis may also occur. Since the introduction of newer, more effective antibiotics, extension of infection is much less common.

Nasal Polyps

Nasal polyps comprise the most common group of mass lesions in the nose. They appear to be outgrowths of the nasal mucosa and are typically smooth, gelatinous, semitranslucent, round or pear shaped, and pale. They are located on the lateral wall of the nose, usually in the middle meatus. Most nasal polyps arise from the ethmoid sinus.

The pathogenesis of nasal polyps is not known, and presently no one theory adequately explains the formation of all nasal polyps. The two theories most frequently mentioned are the allergic and infectious theories. A number of studies have cast great doubt on the importance of allergy in the development of nasal polyps. The incidence of nasal polyps is significantly higher in patients with nonatopic asthma and rhinitis than in those with atopic rhinitis and asthma. In studies of patients admitted for polypectomy, there appears to be no evidence of an increased incidence of allergic disorders; however, there does seem to be an increased association of nasal polyps and asthma. In one large series of patients with nasal polyposis, there was an asthma incidence of 20%. In this same study, 32% of asthmatic patients had nasal polyps.

The association of nasal polyps, bronchial asthma, and aspirin sensitivity has been well described and is referred to as either the *aspirin triad* or *Samter's triad.* Vasomotor rhinitis associated with profuse rhinorrhea generally occurs first in these patients; then intense nasal congestion with the subsequent development of nasal polyps occurs, followed by bronchial asthma, and finally aspirin sensitivity (5).

The major symptoms of patients with nasal polyps are nasal blockage, hyposmia, rhinorrhea, and postnasal drainage. On physical examination, nasal polyps appear rounded or pear-shaped and translucent. They are soft, gelatinous, mobile, insensitive to manipulation, and do not readily bleed.

The major complication of nasal polyps is sinusitis, but there is also a suggestion that chronic sinusitis may result in production of a hyperplastic mucosa, which may then lead to nasal polyps.

The management of nasal polyps may involve both medical and surgical approaches. Corticosteroids are extremely effective in reducing polyp size and can be administered systemically or by aerosol. A wide variety of intranasal preparations of corticosteroids have been shown to be effective in managing nasal polyps. A reasonable medical approach to nasal polyps would be a 10- to 14-day course of oral prednisone, beginning with 60 mg/d in the adult patient and followed by intranasal corticosteroids. In the case of marked mechanical obstruction (particularly with associated sinusitis), polypectomy may have to be performed. Functional endoscopic sinus surgery—a procedure that removes the tissue source of polyps—has been reported to result in a significantly smaller recurrence rate. For many years, controversy has centered on the safety of surgical removal of nasal polyps in patients with asthma and particularly those with intolerance to aspirin. Several carefully controlled studies have shown polypectomy 1) to be safe, 2) to have little effect on the development of asthma, and 3) to have little effect on the bronchial reactivity and severity of asthma once it has been established.

Case 3.2

A 57-year-old physician with a long history of perennial rhinitis developed wheezing for the first time, intensified by exercise and cold air. This was associated with a severe cough at night. After playing tennis one night, he became dyspneic, collapsed, and was hospitalized with severe asthma. In the hospital, he received intensive therapy, including high doses of corticosteroids.

One month later, the patient was still on 20 mg/d of prednisone. Examination of the chest revealed generalized rhonchi and wheezing. The nose showed edematous, erythematous turbinates and mucopus in the nose and posterior pharynx. Chest radiographs showed hyperinflation. Skin tests to common inhalants were negative. Sinus radiographs were positive, showing marked mucoperiosteal thickening and air–fluid levels in the maxillary sinuses.

The patient was treated with amoxicillin, oral decongestants, and nasal steroids, with marked improvement in his clinical state. His chest examination cleared, and his sinus radiographs became normal. One month later, however, he had a recurrence of wheezing. Bilateral nasal antrostomies were performed and revealed massive disease of the maxillary sinuses with large amounts of pus and hyperplastic mucosa. For the next 2 months, despite antibiotics, his purulent drainage continued, as did his wheezing. At that point, functional endoscopic sinus surgery was performed, with marked improvement in nasal, sinus, and chest symptoms.

The patient has continued to do well, with approximately one bout of sinusitis per year. Asthma medications consist only of occasional use of a β-agonist inhaler.

Asthma

The frequent association of nasal and paranasal sinus disease with bronchial asthma was first appreciated many years ago. In recent years, the clinical association of sinusitis and asthma has been revived. A recent study reported abnormal sinus radiographs in 87% of adults, with exacerbation of asthma.

There is no doubt that sinusitis and asthma coexist, but the overriding question is whether sinusitis and asthma are manifestations of the same disease process in different parts of the respiratory tract or whether sinusitis actually triggers bronchial asthma. There are data indicating that patients with refractory asthma show improvement when concurrent sinusitis is appropriately managed, which strongly suggests an etiologic role of sinusitis in lower airway disease (6).

What To Look for When Usual Measures Fail

When a case of sinusitis fails to respond to the usual modes of therapy or if the sinusitis clears only to be followed by a recurrence shortly thereafter, there are four conditions to consider: allergy, immunodeficiency, fungal infection, and structural abnormalities.

Allergy

A number of studies indicate that the incidence of allergy in patients with sinusitis is high. On the other side of the coin, several studies have looked at the incidence of sinusitis in patients with allergic rhinitis, and this figure is also significantly increased. There appears to be a minimum concordance of allergy and sinusitis of 25%, with a maximum concordance of 70%. This is clearly above the general prevalence of allergy and supports the impression that allergy is an important associated and probable predisposing factor in sinusitis.

Immunodeficiency

The following conditions should suggest to the clinician the possibility for immunologic evaluation:
1. Frequent episodes of sinusitis occurring more than three times per year.
2. Failure of appropriate medical management or a return of symptoms less than 1 month after discontinuing antibiotics.
3. Recurrence of sinusitis after surgery.

It should be emphasized that the patient with chronic sinusitis is much more likely to be allergic than immune deficient; therefore, one should do an allergy evaluation before embarking on an extensive immunologic evaluation. The incidence of immune deficiency in chronic sinusitis appears to be significantly higher in children than in adults. An appropriate approach to evaluating immune function is to obtain quantitative immunoglobulins and determine the specific antibody responses to pneumococcal titers before and after immunization and diphtheria or tetanus antibody titers (7).

Fungal Infection

Fungal infection of the sinuses can be divided into four categories: acute/fulminant, chronic/indolent (both of which are examples of invasive sinusitis), fungus ball or mycetoma, and allergic fungal sinusitis. The criteria for the diagnosis of allergic fungal sinusitis are:
1. Sinusitis of one or more paranasal sinuses on imaging.

2. Identification of allergic mucin, which includes the presence of eosinophils and Charcot–Leyden crystals.
3. Demonstration of fungal elements.
4. Absence of diabetes, immunodeficiency diseases, and treatment with immunosuppressive drugs.
5. Absence of invasive fungal disease.

Allergic fungal sinusitis is most common in adolescents and young adults and is associated generally with nasal polyps. Patients characteristically produce brown, rubbery, peanut butter–like nasal plugs. A number of organisms have been shown to be responsible for fungal sinusitis, including *Aspergillus*, *Bipolaris*, *Curvularia*, and *Drechslera*. Diagnosis of allergic fungal sinusitis is made by demonstration of allergic mucin, fungal elements in the nasal smear, and characteristic CT scan showing high-density areas resulting from production of metal elements by the fungi (8).

The treatment of invasive fungal sinusitis consists of extensive debridement and parenteral antifungal drugs. Treatment of allergic fungal sinusitis includes debridement generally by functional endoscopic sinus surgery and an extended course of corticosteroids.

Structural Abnormalities

A number of anatomic problems may account for the failure of chronic sinusitis to respond to medical therapy. These include septal deviation, bone spur, nasal polyps, and ostiomeatal complex obstruction. The therapy of choice, as stated previously, is functional FESS.

When To Refer a Patient with Sinusitis

The vast majority of sinusitis cases can be managed by the primary care physician. Box 3.3 lists those situations for which referral to a specialist is indicated. Figure 3.2 shows an overall diagnostic and therapeutic algorithm.

Box 3.3 When To Refer a Patient with Sinusitis

Recurrent symptoms that interfere with daily activities
Symptoms or infection not controlled by therapy
Recurrent infections in an allergic patient
Sinus disease in association with asthma
Structural abnormalities

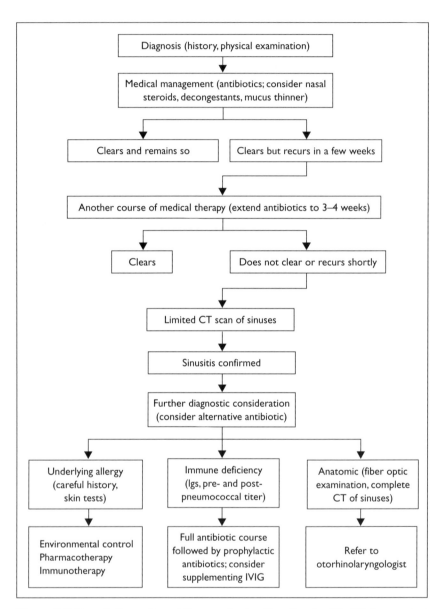

Figure 3.2 Overall diagnostic and therapeutic algorithm for sinusitis. CT = computed tomography; IVIG = intravenous immunoglobulin. (Adapted from Slavin RG. Atlas of Allergies. 2nd ed. St. Louis: Mosby-Wolfe; 1996.)

REFERENCES

1. **Lund VJ, Kennedy DW.** Quantification for staging sinusitis: the staging and therapy group. Ann Otol Rhinol Laryngol. 1995;167(Suppl):17–21.

2. **Milgrim LM, Rubin JS, Rosenstreich DL, Small CB.** Sinusitis in human immuno-deficiency virus infection: typical and atypical organisms. J Otolaryngol. 1994;23: 450–3.

3. **Oliverio PJ, Benson ML, Zinreich SJ.** Update on imaging for functional endoscopic sinus surgery. Otolaryngol Clin North Am. 1995;28:585–608.

4. **Gwaltney JM Jr, Phillips CD, Miller RD, Riker DK.** Computed tomographic study of the common cold. N Eng J Med. 1994;330:25–30.

5. **Settipane GA, Chaffee FJ, Klein DE.** Aspirin intolerance: a prospective study in an atopic and normal population. J Allergy Clin Immunol. 1974;53:200–4.

6. **English GM.** Nasal polypectomy and sinus surgery in patients with asthma and as-pirin idiosyncrasy. Laryngoscopy. 1986;96:374–380.

7. **Polmar S.** The role of the immunologist in sinus disease. J Allergy Clin Immunol. 1992;90:511–5.

8. **de Shazo RD, Swain RZ.** Diagnostic criteria for allergic fungal sinusitis. J Allergy Clin Immunol. 1995;96:24–35.

SUGGESTED READINGS

Kaliner MA, Osguthorpe JD, Fireman P, et al. Sinusitis: bench to bedside. J Allergy Clin Immunol. 1997;99:S829–48.

Slavin RG. Nasal polyps and sinusitis. In: Kaplan A, ed. Allergy. 2nd ed. Philadelphia: WB Saunders; 1997:448–59.

Chapter 4

Asthma

Hiroshi Chantaphakul, MD
William W. Busse, MD

The face of asthma has changed dramatically in the past 20 years. For example, asthma prevalence and severity have significantly increased. Furthermore, the focus of treatment has moved from control of bronchospasm to regulation of inflammation. Although there has been an increase in our understanding of the pathogenesis of asthma and its treatment, asthma remains a common disease for primary care. To achieve optimal care of asthma, it will be helpful to review the presentations of asthma, diagnostic evaluations, differential diagnosis, and management based on disease severity and underlying inflammation.

Definition

Asthma is defined as a disease of variable airway obstruction, chronic inflammation, and airway hyperresponsiveness (Box 4.1) (1). The pathologic findings of asthma include chronic inflammation of the airways in which many cells participate, including mast cells, eosinophils, T lymphocytes, neutrophils, and epithelial cells (2). In the susceptible individual, this inflammatory process can lead to clinical manifestations of asthma, recurrent episodes of wheezing, shortness of breath, chest tightness, and cough, as well as a per-

---

Box 4.1 Definition of Asthma

Airway obstruction with variable reversibility
Chronic inflammation of the airway
Bronchial hyperresponsiveness

---

sistence of disease. These symptoms are associated with abnormalities in pulmonary function—a variable and usually reversible airflow obstruction. Airway hyperresponsiveness, another feature of asthma, likely is caused by airway inflammation, which explains the enhanced susceptibility of the asthmatic airway to undergo bronchial obstruction.

Epidemiology

Asthma affects more than 14 million people in the United States. Although the age of onset of asthma is variable, its peak incidence is 5 years of age. Asthma is the most common chronic disease of childhood, affecting an estimated 4.8 million children, with a worldwide prevalence of childhood asthma ranging from 1.4% to 11.4% (Box 4.2) (3). Asthma is nearly 30% more frequent in prepubescent boys than girls; however, after puberty, the female prevalence increases because asthma affects women more commonly than men. Asthma is not a trivial disease; the National Health Interview Survey reports that asthma in children in the United States accounts for 10.1 million lost school days, 12.9 million extra physician visits, and 200,000 hospitalization per year. In adults, the incidence of asthma ranges from 3.0% to 7.9% with geographic and racial variations. People with asthma collectively have more than 100 million days of restricted activity and 470,000 days of hospitalization annually. During the 1980s, the mortality rate from asthma in the United States increased by 6.2% per year, with the annual age-adjusted death rate for asthma increasing from 13.4 per 1 million to 18.8 per 1 million population from 1982 through 1991. More than 5000 people die of asthma annually in the United States.

Box 4.2 Epidemiology

Asthma prevalence has increased
Asthma onset occurs predominantly but not exclusively in childhood

---

Clinical Presentation

History

Clinical history is an important component of patient evaluation and is critical to making the diagnosis and determining the appropriate level of therapy. Several common presenting symptoms are usually elicited in all patients in whom asthma is considered (Box 4.3). Most patients complain of shortness of breath; this often is associated with wheezing–a high-pitched whistling sound heard or experienced during exhalation. Wheezing is common and occurs particularly during exacerbations or acute episodes of asthma. Recurrent wheezing, difficulty breathing, and chest tightness are common symptoms and appear or increase during exercise, with upper respiratory infections, and following allergen exposure. The presence of these symptoms is suggestive of asthma; however, many patients can have significant airway obstruction and not wheeze or admit to shortness of breath.

Recurrent, nonproductive cough is another characteristic symptom (sometimes the only presenting symptom) of asthma and is particularly troublesome at night. Furthermore, patients often relate that "colds go right to their chest," and they often experience prolonged episodes of coughing at this time. Exercise-induced symptoms of asthma occur in many, if not all, patients with asthma. Shortness of breath, chest tightness, and wheezing may appear during or at the completion of exercise; they can last for several minutes to hours, depending upon the severity of the attack. Consequently, patients with asthma consciously or unconsciously limit their physical activity to prevent the devel-

---

Box 4.3 History

Wheeze, cough, dyspnea, and chest tightness
Symptoms worsen
  At night
  On exertion
  With viral infection
  Following allergen exposure
  With exposure to irritants (smoke, chemical, fume)
Previous treatment
  Response to bronchodilator
  Emergency department visit, hospitalization
  History of respiratory failure
  Need for and response to corticosteroids

opment of such symptoms. Finally, asthma should be suspected in persons with unexplained episodes of dyspnea, cough, repeated "chest cold," or recurrent "bronchitis," especially if they are nonsmokers.

Patients with asthma are particularly prone to symptoms of cough, wheezing, and shortness of breath at night. For example, respiratory arrest and death from asthma are more likely to occur between midnight and 6 AM than at any other time of the day. Furthermore, the frequency of nocturnal awaking (particularly with cough, wheeze, and chest tightness) and the reduction of symptoms with a bronchodilator are helpful in determining the presence and severity of asthma.

Asthma symptoms also worsen with upper respiratory tract infections, which usually are due to viruses. Rhinovirus and influenza virus are the major causes of wheezing in adults. In contrast, respiratory syncytial virus infection is a common cause of wheezing in children. *Mycoplasma pneumoniae* infections often aggravate asthma in adolescent and adult patients. The mechanisms by which viral respiratory infections increase asthma severity have not been fully established. Finally, sinusitis can increase asthma symptoms and severity.

Allergen sensitization is an important risk factor for the development of asthma and asthma exacerbations. Studies have shown that sensitivity to indoor allergens (e.g., house dust mites, cats, and cockroaches) is common in asthma sufferers and likely relates to the development of the disease. Seasonal increases in asthma symptoms occur with exposure to outdoor allergens, such as ragweed, grass, and tree pollens. The mold *Alternaria* is particularly important to the development of asthma. Increases in emergency room visits for acute asthma attack are associated with increases in *Alternaria* exposure during the late summer. The seasonal increase of *Alternaria* has also been considered a major cause of asthma deaths.

Respiratory irritants (e.g., tobacco smoke, strong odors, airborne chemicals, and dust) may also increase asthma symptoms. Exposure to chemicals at work can be a cause of asthma; therefore, a careful evaluation of occupational and recreational exposure is important in the evaluation of asthma.

Asthma often coexists with allergic rhinitis and sinusitis. These conditions can also complicate or trigger the asthma exacerbations and, when brought under control, can improve the asthmatic state. Gastroesophageal reflux disease (GERD) can influence the severity of asthma. Increased abdominal pressure from coughing can aggravate the reflux symptoms and thus establish a vicious cycle of asthma–GERD–asthma. Furthermore, asthma treatment with theophylline decreases lower esophageal sphincter tone, which can then aggravate reflux disease and, hence, asthma. Treatment of GERD may decrease asthma severity.

Other common medical conditions mimic asthma, including coronary artery disease (chest tightness), congestive heart failure (shortness of breath), or emphysema and chronic bronchitis (cough, wheeze, and shortness of breath). For example, a long history of smoking tobacco, productive cough, and recurrent bronchitis suggests chronic obstructive pulmonary disease (COPD) as the cause of shortness of breath rather than asthma. Chest pain with exertion, the presence of palpitations, and edema of the lower extremities are frequent findings of cardiac disease either exclusively or as a coexisting condition. Treatment of comorbid medical conditions may adversely affect asthma; for example, β-adrenergic antagonists for treatment of heart disease or glaucoma can increase asthma severity. Aspirin and other nonsteroidal anti-inflammatory agents can cause asthma exacerbations in aspirin-sensitive persons; asthma attacks associated with aspirin can be severe.

The history should also include a description of the characteristics and pattern of respiratory symptoms. The pattern of the symptoms (e.g., at night, with exercise, during respiratory infection) is as important as frequency, duration, and intensity of symptoms in recognizing asthma and its severity. Marked variability in symptoms can be seen in patients with severe disease. Nighttime awakening, missed days from work or school, and limitation of physical activity are all indicators of more severe asthma or poor asthma control.

It is important to inquire about previous treatment and the response to these approaches as well as about emergency room visits, hospitalizations, or the presence of respiratory failure. The levels of responses to inhaled bronchodilators or systemic corticosteroids are also important clues to the presence and severity of asthma.

A family history of asthma, respiratory allergy, and atopic dermatitis is common in patients with asthma. A detailed history of allergen exposure and its influence on asthma symptoms is helpful. As discussed above, details of seasonal variations of symptoms and aggravation of symptoms during exposure, such as to pets, also should be elicited. In the treatment of an acute attack, it is also important to know the time of onset, the presumed trigger (e.g., respiratory infection, irritant, allergen, work, exercise, cold air, emotions), present medication use, and recent use of corticosteroids. These factors may predict the severity of the disease and the likelihood for response to treatment.

Physical Examination

Physical findings are variable and dependent upon the severity of asthma at the time of examination (Box 4.4). In contrast to the history, which yields a great deal of information in most asthmatic patients, the physical examination in asymptomatic patients is frequently unremarkable. Because airway obstruction is variable and usually reversible, the chest examination during asymptomatic times is likely to be normal. Furthermore, asthma patients tend to do better during the day, and the physical examination can be normal then, even though symptoms are severe at night. With active asthma, there are often inspiratory and expiratory wheezes.

Examination of the upper respiratory tract can provide evidence of coexisting nasal allergy. Mouth breathing, dry or chapped lips, conjunctival injection, suborbital puffiness or bluish discoloration (i.e., "allergic" shiner), furrows of the lower lid (i.e., Dennie–Morgan lines), and retracted tympanic membranes are indicative of allergic rhinitis or atopic dermatitis. The nasal examination may demonstrate a transverse crease over the bridge, especially in children, caused by the frequent rubbing of the nose to relieve nasal itching. The nasal turbinates are pale and edematous with coexisting allergic rhinitis. The presence of nasal polyps suggests the possibility of coexisting sinusitis or aspirin sensitivity; cystic fibrosis is another cause of nasal polyps. The posterior pharynx may show postnasal mucosal drainage or "cobblestoning" due to retropharyngeal lymphoid hyperplasia. Inspiratory stridor suggests consideration of upper airway obstruction or conditions such as vocal cord dysfunction as a cause of wheezing. An abnormal third heart sound or cardiac murmur raises the possibility that cardiac disease is the cause of symptoms rather than asthma. The skin and extremities examination may reveal evidence of atopic dermatitis. Digital clubbing does not occur in asthma and suggests other chronic obstructive pulmonary disease, cardiac problem, or cystic fibrosis.

With active or severe asthma, wheezing is the most common finding on auscultation of the chest. Loud wheezing during both inspiration and expiration is associated with more significant airflow obstruction; however, it is important to remember that wheezing may be absent in very severe airway obstruction or during severe asthma attack because of a marked limitation to airflow. Hyperexpansion of the thoracic cage may be obvious, especially in children, and results from an adaptive response to the breathing against the narrowed airway. The use of accessory muscles, a prolonged expiratory phase, and a barrel-shaped chest are other physical findings associated with chronic asthma or with a severe exacerbation.

In severe asthma, patients are often agitated, anxious, fatigued, somnolent, and have interrupted speech and the need to sit in an upright position. Vital

---

Box 4.4 Physical Examination

Possibly normal during asymptomatic periods
Wheezing with greater airway obstruction
Thorax hyperexpansion
Signs of coexisting allergic rhinitis or atopic dermatitis

signs reveal tachypnea, tachycardia, and hypertension; in severe cases, a pulsus paradoxus greater than 15 mm Hg is frequently a finding. Nasal flaring, use of accessory muscles of respiration, thorax overinflation, prolonged expiration, and diffuse inspiratory and expiratory wheezing are also obvious with acute, severe asthma. When acute episodes of asthma lead to impending respiratory failure, the patients may be cyanotic and have asterixis, severe respiratory distress, confusion, somnolence, and diaphoresis. In very severe asthma with a marked reduction in airflow, breath sounds are often inaudible or distant.

Risk Factors for Increases in Asthma Mortality

Significant risk factors for severe asthma or even death include a previous history of life-threatening asthma, respiratory arrest, or hospitalization in the past year. Patients who have a poor perception of existing hypoxia or sudden, severe airflow obstruction are also at risk for fatal episodes. Elderly patients as well as adolescents who have poor asthma control are at greater risk for death from asthma. Patients with *Alternaria* allergy have a higher incidence of emergency room visits and death during late summer. Psychologic disturbances, including depression and family dysfunction, heighten the risk of fatal asthma (Box 4.5).

Diagnosis and Classification of Asthma Severity

The diagnosis of asthma is based upon history, physical examination, and objective measurement of lung function. The information from the patient's history and findings on physical examination are both important to the diagnosis

---

Box 4.5 Risks Factors for Fatal Asthma

Adolescent and elderly persons

Previous history of severe asthma exacerbation, requiring intensive care or causing respiratory failure

Poor perception of hypoxia, airway obstruction, or both

Overuse of inhaled bronchodilator

Psychologic factor

Allergy to *Alternaria* mold

Recent withdrawal from corticosteroids

of asthma. The measurement of lung function, however, is helpful and essential to make the diagnosis of asthma and to follow the patient's response to treatment. Approximately two thirds of asthma patients and their physicians cannot predict their lung function based on a perception of current symptoms. There appears to be a trend toward underdiagnosis and underestimation of asthma severity. Consequently, patients whose history and physical findings suggest asthma should be evaluated with an objective measurement of pulmonary function (Box 4.6).

Spirometry is commonly used in clinical practice and is effective to establish the level of airflow obstruction. The most precise measurement of airflow obstruction is the forced expiratory volume in one second (FEV_1). This value should be compared with the forced expiratory volume (or forced vital capacity [FVC]) to determine whether there is an obstructive or restrictive pattern to the lung functions. In severe asthma, the FVC is often reduced, giving the appearance of a coexisting restrictive pattern. Consequently, there is often a reduction both in the FVC and FEV_1 in moderate to severe asthma. Measurements of peak expiratory flow with a peak-flow meter also provide a quick and simple means of monitoring lung function.

For the patients with active asthma, spirometry should be repeated after a bronchodilator (e.g., inhaled β-adrenergic agonist) to determine if there is an increase in FEV_1, usually more than 12% or an absolute improvement of 200 mL (4,5). Such a response indicates reversibility of airway obstruction, a finding compatible with asthma. The airway response to a bronchodilator can be suboptimal in patients with more severe disease or obstruction. This does not necessarily mean that they do not have asthma but rather that a component of their airflow obstruction is secondary to bronchial inflammation and not bronchospasm alone. To improve lung function in the face of bronchial inflammation, it is sometimes helpful to administer a short course (7–10 d) of oral corticosteroids (e.g., prednisone 10 mg tid for the first 5 d,

---

Box 4.6 Evaluation of Asthmatic Patients

History and physical examination

Spirometry necessary to make objective measurements of the airway obstruction and follow response to treatment

Provocation test for airway hyperresponsiveness with normal lung function

Arterial blood gas determinations in severe airflow obstruction or pending respiratory failure

Chest radiograph, complete blood count, and electrolytes may be helpful with coexisting treatment or other diseases

followed by 10 mg qd for 5 d or 1 mg/kg/d in divided dose for children). Oral corticosteroids can reduce inflammation and improve pulmonary functions if asthma exists.

In patients whose history is characteristic or suggestive of asthma, but who have normal lung function on spirometry, the demonstration of bronchial hyperresponsiveness with provocation testing is helpful in diagnosing an airway feature compatible with asthma. Methacholine provocation consists of having patients inhale an aerosolized cholinergic agonist. If airway hyperresponsiveness exists, airway bronchoconstriction will occur at low doses of these agents. Approximately 95% of asthmatic patients have a bronchial hyperresponsiveness to methacholine. A heightened bronchoconstrictive response to methacholine (or bronchial hyperresponsiveness) is not diagnostic of asthma but rather compatible with the disease. Bronchial hyperresponsiveness is also found in patients with allergic rhinitis, COPD, congestive heart failure, cystic fibrosis, or following a recent viral respiratory infection. A decrease in FEV_1 of 20% to inhaled methacholine or more is a positive response. Patients who have significant airway obstruction (i.e., $FEV_1 < 70\%$) are at risk for severe episodes of bronchospasm with inhaled methacholine and should not receive this test. The methacholine challenge testing should be performed by physicians who are trained and experienced in this technique.

During an acute exacerbation of asthma, all patients should have spirometry or measures of peak expiratory flow to define a more precise degree of bronchial obstruction. These measurements aid in the diagnosis of acute asthma, determine its severity, and serve as a monitor to treatment. Arterial blood gas determinations are helpful in the management of patients with severe respiratory distress, impending respiratory failure, or in patients with a history of respiratory failure. In moderately severe asthma, there is compensatory hyperventilation, and this is reflected in arterial blood gas determinants, which show hypocapnia, hypoxia, and respiratory alkalosis. As airflow obstruction becomes more severe, hypoxia is more profound; carbon dioxide retention occurs from muscle fatigue and the progressive worsening of airway obstruction, which leads to a furthering of the ventilation–perfusion mismatch. Patients with these signs of impending respiratory failure should be admitted to an intensive care unit, because they have high risk for respiratory failure and need close monitoring and aggressive treatment.

Chest radiography may be helpful in diagnosing pneumonia, pneumothorax, or congestive heart failure, but it is not indicated for all asthma patients. A complete blood count can show an elevation of the eosinophil count in patients with more severe asthma. Leukocytosis may present in patients who are receiving systemic corticosteroid or in patients with a coexisting infection. Hypokalemia from dehydration, corticosteroid treatment, and bronchodilator treatment may be found in these patients.

Differential Diagnosis

The differential diagnosis of asthma in adults (Box 4.7) includes congestive heart failure, especially pulmonary edema, which can present with acute respiratory distress and wheezing. A history and other findings of cardiac disease (e.g., crackles or rales in the chest or a third heart sound on auscultation) will help distinguish this condition from asthma. COPD (e.g., chronic bronchitis, emphysema, and bronchiectasis) can mimic asthma. Chronic bronchitis and emphysema are most often associated with a long history of tobacco smoking. The clinical presentation for COPD is variable and includes chronic cough, dyspnea on exertion, or both. The response to bronchodilators is usually min-

---

Box 4.7 Differential Diagnosis

Other pulmonary disorders
> Chronic obstructive pulmonary disease
> Pulmonary embolism
> Pulmonary infiltration and eosinophilia
> Interstitial lung disease
> Viral bronchiolitis
> Obliterative bronchiolitis
> Bronchopulmonary dysplasia
> α-1 antiprotease deficiency
> Cystic fibrosis

Cough secondary to medication
> Angiotensin-converting-enzyme inhibitor
> Large airway diseases
> Vocal cord dysfunction
> Vascular rings
> Laryngeal web
> Laryngotracheomalacia
> Foreign body
> Enlarged lymph nodes or tumor

Cardiovascular conditions
> Congestive heart failure
> Ischemic heart disease

Psychologic conditions
> Hyperventilation syndrome
> Panic attack

imal. These conditions co-exist in asthma, and a more detailed study of pulmonary function (which may demonstrate restrictive pattern on abnormal diffusing capacity) and chest radiographic studies are usually necessary to assist in making the correct diagnosis. Other less common conditions, such as tumors of the tracheobronchial tree, can mimic asthma by obstructing the airway enough to cause wheezing, chronic cough, and progressive dyspnea as the tumor grows.

Patients with vocal cord dysfunction—a paradoxical adduction of the vocal cords during inspiration—present with symptoms that mimic asthma, including inspiratory dyspnea and wheezing. These symptoms usually do not occur at night and do not improve with bronchodilators. The pulmonary function test is often disproportionately abnormal in relationship to the severity of symptoms. An inspiratory "cut-off" may be seen on the inspiratory flow volume loop when the patient is symptomatic with vocal cord dysfunction. Direct visualization of the vocal cords while the patient is symptomatic can demonstrate a paradoxical movement of the vocal cord during inspiration—the gold standard for the diagnosis. Vocal cord dysfunction can occur in association with asthma in up to 30% of patients.

Treatment

Successful management of asthma patients requires an understanding of basic treatment principles. As previously discussed, asthma is a chronic inflammatory disorder of the airway, with recurrent episodes of wheezing, breathlessness, chest tightness, and coughing. The primary principle of treatment is to suppress inflammation, normalize lung function, and prevent exacerbations.

The aim of asthma therapy is to maintain control of asthma with the least amount of medication, thus minimizing the possibilities for adverse effects from drugs. The Expert Panel on Asthma Management has suggested the goals for asthma treatment listed in Box 4.8 (1).

Pharmacologic therapy is now categorized into two general classes: quick-relief and long-term–control medications (Box 4.9). Quick-relief medications are designed to control the acute symptoms and include short-acting β_2-adrenergic agonist, anticholinergics, and systemic corticosteroids. Long-term–control medications are used on a regular basis and include corticosteroid inhalers or tablets, cromolyn sodium and necrodomil sodium inhalers, long-acting β_2-agonists, methylxanthines, and leukotriene modifiers. Although many of the long-term control medications have an anti-inflammatory effect, this is not true for all. These medications are defined by how they are used.

Short-acting β_2-adrenergic agonists (e.g., albuterol, bitolterol, pirbuterol, and terbutaline) are effective for quick relief of acute bronchospasm. They re-

---

Box 4.8 Goals for Asthma Treatment

To prevent chronic and troublesome symptoms (e.g., cough or breathlessness at
night, in the early morning, or after exertion)
To maintain normal (or near normal) pulmonary function
To maintain normal activity levels
To prevent recurrent exacerbations of asthma and minimize the need for emer-
gency department visits or hospitalizations
To provide optimal pharmacotherapy with minimal or no adverse effects
To meet patients' and families' expectations of and satisfaction with asthma care

Data from National Heart, Lung, and Blood Institute Guidelines for the Diagnosis and
Management of Asthma. Bethesda, MD: National Institutes of Health; 1997; NIH Publication No. 97-4051.

---

lax airway smooth muscle and cause, in many cases, a prompt increase in airflow. Inhaled β_2-agonists are the therapy of choice for control of acute asthma
symptoms and also to prevent exercise-induced bronchospasm. They are
available in both inhaler and solution form for use in a nebulizer (Table 4.1).
The oral forms of short-acting β_2-adrenergic agonist are not effective for
quick relief.

Anticholinergics such as ipratropium bromide (a quaternary derivative
of atropine with less cholinergic side effect) provide an additional benefit
when used with inhaled β_2-adrenergic agonists in severe exacerbation (*see*
Table 4.1).

Systemic corticosteroids (i.e., prednisone, prednisolone, and methylprednisolone) are used in episodes of moderate-to-severe asthma exacerbations to
improve airflow obstruction in acute asthma that does not respond to quick
relief from β_2-agonists (Figs. 4.1 and 4.2 and Table 4.1). The early use of high-
dose systemic corticosteroids during severe exacerbation controls the inflammation and thus improves airflow limitation.

The long-term–control medications, especially those with anti-inflammatory actions, are the most important and effective treatment of persistent
asthma. Of the anti-inflammatory medications, corticosteroids are the most
potent and effective (Table 4.2). Corticosteroids decrease bronchial hyperresponsiveness, improve lung function, and prevent asthma exacerbations.

The long-acting inhaled β_2-agonist salmeterol is most commonly used concomitantly with anti-inflammatory medication and, under these conditions,
provides an additional benefit (6). At present there is no evidence that inhaled
long-acting β_2-agonists have anti-inflammatory effects. Consequently, it is recommended that inhaled long-acting β_2-agonists be used with corticosteroids.

Box 4.9 Pharmacologic Classifications of Treatment for Asthma

Quick-relief medications
  Inhaled short-acting β_2-adrenergic agonists
    Albuterol
    Bitolterol
    Pirbuterol
    Terbutaline
  Anticholinergics
    Ipratropium
  Systemic corticosteroids
    Prednisone
    Prednisolone
    Methylprednisolone
Long-term control medications
  Inhaled corticosteroids
    Beclomethasone dipropionate
    Budesonide Turbuhaler
    Flunisolide
    Fluticasone
    Triamcinolone acetonide
  Systemic corticosteroids
    Prednisolone
    Prednisone
    Methylprednisolone
  Cromolyn sodium and necrodomil inhalers
  Long-acting β_2-agonists
    Salmeterol inhaler
  Methylxanthines
    Theophylline
  Leukotriene modifiers
    Montelukast
    Zafirlukast
    Zileuton

Cromolyn sodium and necrodomil sodium have modest anti-inflammatory effects; nonetheless, they are often used as initial long-term–control therapy in children because of their safety record. Cromolyn sodium can also be used before exercise or exposure to unavoidable aeroallergens to prevent increased asthma under these circumstances. Their use is particularly helpful, for exam-

Table 4.1 Usual Dosages of Quick-Relief Medications

Medication	Dose Form	Dose	Adult Dosage
Short-acting inhaled β$_2$-agonists			
Albuterol	MDI	90 μg/puff	2 puffs 5 min before
Albuterol HFA	MDI	90 μg/puff	exercise, 2 puffs
Bitolterol	MDI	370 μg/puff	tid–qid, or both
Pirbuterol	MDI	200 μg/puff	
Terbutaline	MDI	200 μg/puff	
Albuterol rotahaler	DPI	200 μg/capsule	1–2 capsules q 4–6 h as needed and before exercise
Albuterol	Nebulizer solution	5 μg/mL (0.5%)	1.25–5.00 mg (0.25–1.00 cm³) in 2–3 cm³ of saline q 4–8 h
Bitolterol	Nebulizer solution	2 μg/mL (0.2%)	0.5–3.5 mg (0.25–1.00 cm³) in 2–3 cm³ of saline q 4–8 h
Anticholinergics			
Ipratropium	MDI	18 μg/puff	2–3 puffs q 6 h
	Nebulizer solution	0.25 mg/mL (0.025%)	0.25–0.5 mg q 6 h
Systemic corticosteroids			
Methylprednisolone	Tablets	2, 4, 8, 32 mg	Short course "burst":
Prednisolone	Tablets	5 mg	40–60 mg/d as single or
	Nebulizer solution	5, 15 mg/cm³	2 divided doses for 3–10 d
Prednisone	Tablets	1, 2.5, 5, 10, 20, 25 mg	
	Nebulizer solution	5 mg/cm³	

DPI = dry-powdered inhaler; MDI = metered-dose inhaler.
Modified from National Heart, Lung, and Blood Institute Guidelines for the Diagnosis and Management of Asthma. Bethesda, MD: National Institutes of Health; 1997; NIH Publication No. 97-4051.

ple, with animal exposure, such as might occur with patients who periodically visit relatives with furry pets.

Methylxanthines have mild bronchodilator activity and are principally used as adjuvants with inhaled corticosteroids in the treatment of asthma. For some patients, 24-hour, sustained-release theophylline is effective in preventing nocturnal symptoms. Although the mechanism of action for theophylline has yet to be fully established, theophylline has mild anti-inflammatory effects. Monitoring serum concentrations of theophylline is essential to ensure that therapeutic (but not toxic) levels are achieved.

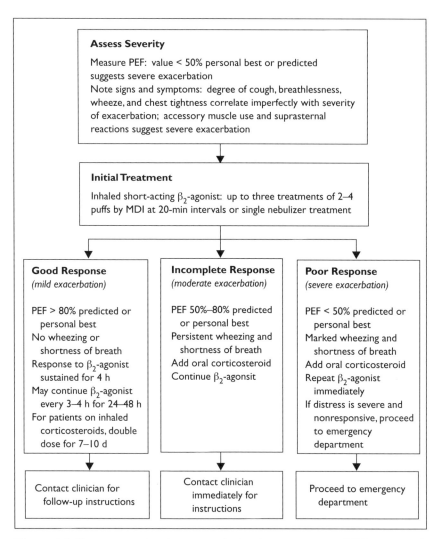

Assess Severity

Measure PEF: value < 50% personal best or predicted suggests severe exacerbation

Note signs and symptoms: degree of cough, breathlessness, wheeze, and chest tightness correlate imperfectly with severity of exacerbation; accessory muscle use and suprasternal reactions suggest severe exacerbation

Initial Treatment

Inhaled short-acting β_2-agonist: up to three treatments of 2–4 puffs by MDI at 20-min intervals or single nebulizer treatment

Good Response
(mild exacerbation)

PEF > 80% predicted or personal best
No wheezing or shortness of breath
Response to β_2-agonist sustained for 4 h
May continue β_2-agonist every 3–4 h for 24–48 h
For patients on inhaled corticosteroids, double dose for 7–10 d

Incomplete Response
(moderate exacerbation)

PEF 50%–80% predicted or personal best
Persistent wheezing and shortness of breath
Add oral corticosteroid
Continue β_2-agonsit

Poor Response
(severe exacerbation)

PEF < 50% predicted or personal best
Marked wheezing and shortness of breath
Add oral corticosteroid
Repeat β_2-agonist immediately
If distress is severe and nonresponsive, proceed to emergency department

Contact clinician for follow-up instructions

Contact clinician immediately for instructions

Proceed to emergency department

Figure 4.1 Management of asthma exacerbation: home treatment. MDI = metered-dose inhaler; PEF = peak expiratory flow. (Adapted from National Heart, Lung, and Blood Institute. Guidelines for the Diagnosis and Management of Asthma. Bethesda, MD: National Institutes of Health; 1997; NIH Publication No. 97-4051.)

Leukotriene modifiers (i.e., zafirlukast, zileuton, and montelukast) may be considered alternative therapy in mild persistent asthma (*see* Box 4.9). These compounds interfere with the actions of leukotrienes and achieve this action either by blocking the leukotriene D_4 receptor (zafirlukast, montelukast) or in-

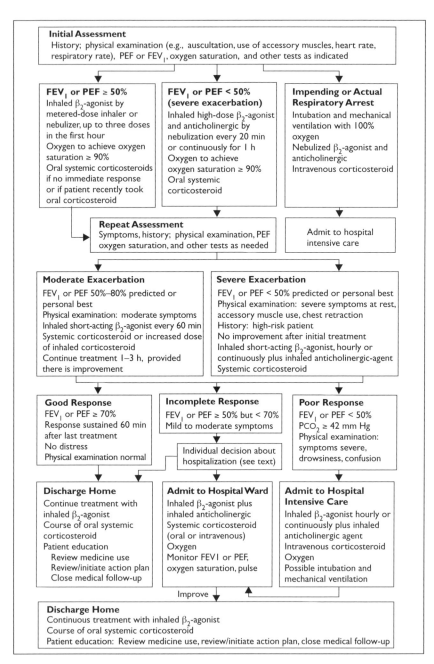

Initial Assessment
History; physical examination (e.g., auscultation, use of accessory muscles, heart rate, respiratory rate), PEF or FEV_1, oxygen saturation, and other tests as indicated

FEV_1 or PEF ≥ 50%
Inhaled β_2-agonist by metered-dose inhaler or nebulizer, up to three doses in the first hour
Oxygen to achieve oxygen saturation ≥ 90%
Oral systemic corticosteroids if no immediate response or if patient recently took oral corticosteroid

FEV_1 or PEF < 50% (severe exacerbation)
Inhaled high-dose β_2-agonist and anticholinergic by nebulization every 20 min or continuously for 1 h
Oxygen to achieve oxygen saturation ≥ 90%
Oral systemic corticosteroid

Impending or Actual Respiratory Arrest
Intubation and mechanical ventilation with 100% oxygen
Nebulized β_2-agonist and anticholinergic
Intravenous corticosteroid

Repeat Assessment
Symptoms, history; physical examination, PEF oxygen saturation, and other tests as needed

Admit to hospital intensive care

Moderate Exacerbation
FEV_1 or PEF 50%–80% predicted or personal best
Physical examination: moderate symptoms
Inhaled short-acting β_2-agonist every 60 min
Systemic corticosteroid or increased dose of inhaled corticosteroid
Continue treatment 1–3 h, provided there is improvement

Severe Exacerbation
FEV_1 or PEF < 50% predicted or personal best
Physical examination: severe symptoms at rest, accessory muscle use, chest retraction
History: high-risk patient
No improvement after initial treatment
Inhaled short-acting β_2-agonist, hourly or continuously plus inhaled anticholinergic-agent
Systemic corticosteroid

Good Response
FEV_1 or PEF ≥ 70%
Response sustained 60 min after last treatment
No distress
Physical examination normal

Incomplete Response
FEV_1 or PEF ≥ 50% but < 70%
Mild to moderate symptoms

Individual decision about hospitalization (see text)

Poor Response
FEV_1 or PEF < 50%
PCO_2 ≥ 42 mm Hg
Physical examination: symptoms severe, drowsiness, confusion

Discharge Home
Continue treatment with inhaled β_2-agonist
Course of oral systemic corticosteroid
Patient education
    Review medicine use
    Review/initiate action plan
    Close medical follow-up

Admit to Hospital Ward
Inhaled β_2-agonist plus inhaled anticholinergic
Systemic corticosteroid (oral or intravenous)
Oxygen
Monitor FEV1 or PEF, oxygen saturation, pulse

Admit to Hospital Intensive Care
Inhaled β_2-agonist hourly or continuously plus inhaled anticholinergic agent
Intravenous corticosteroid
Oxygen
Possible intubation and mechanical ventilation

Improve

Discharge Home
Continuous treatment with inhaled β_2-agonist
Course of oral systemic corticosteroid
Patient education: Review medicine use, review/initiate action plan, close medical follow-up

Figure 4.2 Management of asthma exacerbation: emergency department treatment. FEV_1 = forced expiratory volume in 1 s; PEF = peak expiratory flow; PCO_2 = carbon dioxide partial pressure. (Adapted from National Heart, Lung, and Blood Institute. Guidelines for the Diagnosis and Management of Asthma. Bethesda, MD: National Institutes of Health; 1997; NIH Publication No. 97-4051.)

Table 4.2 Comparative Daily Dosages for Inhaled Corticosteroids

Drug	Low dose	Medium dose	High dose
Beclomethasone dipropionate	168–504 µg	504–840 µg	> 840 µg
42 µg/puff	(4–12 puffs of 42 µg)	(12–20 puffs of 42 µg)	(> 20 puffs of 42 µg)
84 µg/puff	(2–6 puffs of 84 µg)	(6–10 puffs of 84 µg)	(> 10 puffs of 84 µg)
Budesonide Turbuhaler	200–400 µg	400–600 µg	> 600 µg
200 µg/puff	(1–2 inhalations)	(2–3 inhalations)	(> 3 inhalations)
Flunisolide	500–1000 µg	1000–2000 µg	> 2000 µg
250 µg/puff	(2–4 puffs)	(4–8 puffs)	(> 8 puffs)
Fluticasone	88–264 µg	264–660 µg	> 660 µg
MDI: 44, 110, 220 µg/puff	(2–6 puffs of 44 µg; 2 puffs of 110 µg)	(2–6 puffs of 110 µg)	(> 6 puffs of 110 µg; > 3 puffs of 220 µg)
DPI: 50, 100, 250 µg/dose	(2–6 inhalations of 50 µg)	(3–6 inhalations of 100 µg)	(> 6 inhalations of 100 µg; > 2 inhalations of 250 µg)
Triamcinolone acetonide 100 µg/puff	400–1000 µg (4–10 puffs)	1000–2000 µg (10–20 puffs)	> 2000 µg (> 20 puffs)

DPI = dry-powdered inhaler; MDI = metered-dose inhaler.
Modified with permission from National Heart, Lung, and Blood Institute Highlights of the Expert Panel Report 2: Guidelines for the Diagnosis and Management of Asthma. Bethesda, MD. National Institutes of Health: 1997. NIH Publication 97-4051A.

hibiting the 5-lipoxygenase enzyme (zileuton); however, further studies are needed to establish more fully their role in asthma management (1).

The National Heart, Lung, and Blood Institute guidelines have classified asthma into four arbitrary levels according to the clinical presentation and disease severity before treatment. Based on this level of asthma severity, there are treatment guidelines for each group (Table 4.3).

Case 4.1

A 19-year-old female college student had a cough following a basketball practice. These symptoms were present for the past 6 months. She also had experienced shortness of breath following a recent upper respiratory infection, but she was otherwise healthy. Her past history included seasonal allergic rhinitis. She was not taking any medication, and she had never smoked cigarettes.   *Continued*

Case 4.1 (continued)

The physical examination was unremarkable. Sprirometry revealed the following:

	Baseline	Excercise	Postbronchodilator
FEV₁	90% predicted	79% predicted	94% predicted
	3.50 L	2.90 L	3.65 L
FEV₁/FVC	79%	70%	82%

The patient was diagnosed as having mild intermittent asthma, with episodic symptoms due to airflow obstruction that is reversible with bronchodilator. An inhaled bronchodilator was recommended for use before exercise and during viral respiratory infections. During follow-up visit, she reported that she feels better and can participate in basketball practice without a recurrence of symptoms.

Patients with *intermittent* asthma have infrequent symptoms. Furthermore, their symptoms normally are controlled with β-adrenergic bronchodilators as needed. Intermittent asthma does not, however, mean that the asthma that occurs during an exacerbation is always mild. Patients with intermittent asthma can have severe, sudden asthma attacks and then be absolutely symptom free between these attacks. Such episodes often require a "burst" of systemic corticosteroids to achieve control.

Table 4.3 Classification of Severity from the Clinical Presentation

Classification of Severity	Symptoms	Nocturnal Symptoms	Lung Function
Intermittent	2 times per week	≤ 2 times per month	FEV₁ or PEF ≥ 80% predicted
	Asymptomatic between the exacerbation		PEF variability < 20%
Mild persistent	> 2 times per week but < 1 time per day	≥ 2 times per month	FEV₁ or PEF ≥ 80% predicted
	Exacerbation may affect activity	> 1 time per week	PEF variability 20%–30%
Moderate persistent	Daily symptoms	Frequent	FEV₁ or PEF > 60% ≤ 80% predicted
	Exacerbation affect activity		
	Exacerbations ≥ 2 times a week and may last days		PEF variability > 30%
Severe persistent	Continual symptoms		FEV₁ or PEF ≤ 60% predicted
	Limited physical activity		
	Frequent exacerbations		PEF variability > 30%

FEV₁ = forced expiratory volume in 1 s; PEF = peak expiratory flow.
Modified from National Heart, Lung, and Blood Institute Guidelines for the Diagnosis and Management of Asthma. Bethesda, MD: National Institutes of Health; 1997; NIH Publication No. 97-4051.

Case 4.2

A 42-year-old man presented to the emergency room complaining of progressive dyspnea and wheezing that did not improve with the use of an inhaled bronchodilator. He also indicated that he had a cold for the past week. As an adolescent, he had asthma, which reappeared almost 5 years ago. He used theophylline intermittently and took small doses of inhaled corticosteroids. Recently, his albuterol use had been 10 to 12 puffs per day (2 canisters per month). Also, in the past 6 months, he had awakened at least three nights per week with tightness in his chest.

Physical examination revealed a body temperature of 37°C, a pulse of 98 bpm, a respiratory rate of 16 per min., and a blood pressure of 150 over 90. His nasal mucous membranes were reddened, but there was no rhinorrhea. Lung auscultation revealed bilateral and diffuse wheezing. Spirometry revealed the following:

	Baseline	**Postbronchodilator**
FEV_1	55% predicted	
	2.1 L	2.4 L (14% improved)
FEV_1/FVC	50%	

The patient was diagnosed as having moderate to severe persistent asthma, with an acute exacerbation.

Treatment with oral prednisone was recommended, with short-acting β_2-agonist continued as needed.

At one-week follow-up, his condition had markedly improved. He could sleep through the night, and his albuterol use decreased during the past 3 days. The physical examination was within normal limits. His spirometry revealed an FEV_1 of 2.8 L (73% predicted) and an FEV_1/FVC of 70%. He was started on high doses of inhaled corticosteroids, given a peak flow meter, and scheduled for a return visit in 1 month.

Persistent asthma is divided into mild, moderate, and severe. This division is based on the frequency of symptoms, nocturnal awakening from asthma, and level of lung function (*see* Table 4.3). Persistent asthma is most effectively controlled with daily long-term–control medications, which have anti-inflammatory effects. Of the inflammatory compounds, inhaled corticosteroids are the most potent and effective.

The amount and frequency of medication for a particular patient is dictated by the interval history and the level of asthma severity when evaluated (Box 4.10). Although the guidelines were written for "step-care" treatment, therapy is often initiated at a higher level (or "step up") to obtain prompt control of the disease. When patients are stable, treatments are "stepped down." For example, the asthma patient with weekly symptoms of cough, wheeze, and nocturnal awakening initially can be well controlled either by a medium-

---

Box 4.10 Summary of the Management of Asthma

Principle: control airway inflammation

Medication classifications

    Quick-relief medications

    Long-term–control medications

Treatment recommendation depends on asthma severity

    Intermittent asthma

    Persistent asthma (mild, moderate, and severe)

"Step-care" approach and periodic evaluation with "step up" or "step down"

Treatment of acute exacerbation

    Home or emergency department

    Early control of inflammation by systemic steroid

---

to high-dose inhaled corticosteroid (*see* Table 4.2) or a short course of oral prednisone (10 mg tid for 5–7 d). The step-up approach often leads to a more prompt control of asthma symptoms. When patient symptoms are controlled and pulmonary function tests improve, medications can be decreased (or stepped down) to a dose that continues to control symptoms and lung function. This approach is based on the assumption that airway inflammation is more likely to be controlled with an initial higher dose of corticosteroids.

Follow-up visits at intervals of 1 to 6 months are essential to ensure symptom control and an appropriate step up or step down in therapy as indicated (Table 4.4). The frequency of these visits is dictated by disease severity and the patient's response to treatment. The control of active asthma is usually achieved within 1 month of initial therapy if the starting dose of medication is sufficiently high. The patient's pharmacologic management plan should be then re-evaluated at each visit and stepped up or down, depending upon the level of asthma control.

In clinically stable patients with normal or near normal spirometry values at follow-up visits, a step down in the treatment should be considered. The step down in therapy is helpful to identify the minimum level of medication necessary to maintain symptom control and to minimize adverse effects of the drugs.

Although the recommendations are presented as a step-care approach, an individual patient's disease severity may change over time. For example, some patients may experience complete remission of their symptoms during adolescence only to have their asthma recur in greater severity during adulthood. Patients, therefore, should be monitored on a regular basis, and their treatment should be modified to their current condition and medication requirements. Patients should also be counseled that with a return of symptoms, asthma therapy will need to be modified or reinstated.

Table 4.4 Step-wise Approach for Managing Asthma in Adults and Children Over 5 Years of Age*

Classification of Severity	Long-term Control	Quick Relief
Intermittent (step 1)	No daily medication needed	Short-acting bronchodilator: **inhaled β_2-agonists** as needed Intensity of treatment depends on severity of exacerbation Use of β_2-agonists > 2 times a week may indicate need to initiate long-term–control medications
Mild persistent (step 2)	Daily medication: Either **anti-inflammatory inhaled corticosteroid** (low dose) or **cromolyn** or **necrodomil** (in children) Sustained-release theophylline is an alternative; zafirlukast and zileuton may also be considered for patients ≥ 12 years of age	Short-acting bronchodilator: **inhaled β_2-agonists** as needed Intensity of treatment depends on severity of exacerbation Use of β_2-agonists on a daily basis, or increasing use, indicates need for additional long-term–control medications
Moderate persistent (step 3)	Daily medication: Either Anti-inflammatory inhaled corticosteroid (medium dose) *or* Inhaled corticosteroid (low-medium dose) with long-acting bronchodilator **long-acting inhaled β_2-agonist**, sustained-release theophylline, or long-acting β_2-agonists tablets If needed Anti-inflammatory inhaled corticosteroid (medium-high dose) *and* Long-acting bronchodilator, especially for nighttime symptoms; either long-acting inhaled β_2-agonist, sustained-release theophylline, or long-acting β_2-agonists tablets	Short-acting bronchodilator: **inhaled β_2-agonists** as needed Intensity of treatment depends on severity of exacerbation Use of β_2-agonists on a daily basis, or increasing use, indicates need for additional long-term–control medications
Severe persistent (step 4)	Daily medications: **Anti-inflammatory inhaled corticosteroid** (high dose) *and* Long-acting bronchodilator: either long-acting inhaled β_2-agonist, sustained-release theophylline, or long-acting β_2-agonists tablets *and* Corticosteroid tablets or syrup long term (2 mg/kg/d, generally do not exceed 60 mg/d)	Short-acting bronchodilator: **inhaled β_2-agonists** as needed Intensity of treatment depends on severity of exacerbation Use of β_2-agonists on a daily basis, or increasing use, indicates need for additional long-term–control medications

*Treatments of choice are in bold face.

Nonpharmacologic management is also essential to achieve better control of asthma. Avoidance and control of specific triggers (e.g., allergens and smoking) are a major component of asthma management. Furthermore, the more patients understand their disease and the treatment involved, the more likely they will be to adhere to a treatment plan. This approach will increase the success rate of treatment; therefore, all patients should receive asthma education, understand the principles of self- or co-management, and be given an action plan for acute exacerbations (*see* Management of Acute Exacerbations of Asthma).

Case 4.3

A 50-year-old woman with a 10-year history of asthma presented with symptoms that progressively increased over the past 3 years. She had daily asthma attacks and needed to use her albuterol inhaler every 4 hours. She had awakened with cough five to six nights per week and frequently missed work. Her cough and wheeze were worse with any exertion. She was hospitalized twice for an asthma exacerbation with a respiratory infection. At her last admission, she required observation in an intensive-care unit for 2 days because of a severe airflow obstruction. She was never intubated. She was on inhaled triamcinolone (4 puffs twice daily) and salmeterol (2 puffs twice daily).

Physical examination revealed bilateral end expiratory wheeze on lung auscultation. Spirometry revealed

	Baseline	Postbronchodilator
FEV_1	50% predicted	
	1.9 L	2.0 L (5% improved)
FEV_1/FVC	50%	

The patient was diagnosed with severe persistent asthma. Prednisone (40 mg/d in divided doses) was prescribed, and a follow-up visit was scheduled in 1 week. Spirometry revealed an FEV_1 of 2.7 L (70% predicted) and FEV_1/FVC of 65%.

One week later, she felt slightly improved. Her albuterol use was decreased to 3 times per day, and her nighttime waking was also decreased (to once per week). The inhaled corticosteroid was changed to fluticasone (880 µg/d), and the prednisone was gradually tapered. Her asthma symptoms recurred when her prednisone was reduced below 5 mg/d. It was recommended that she continue with low-dose prednisone (5 mg/d) as well as inhaled corticosteroids and an inhaled long-acting $beta_2$-agonist.

At a subsequent 4-week follow-up, the patient felt better. She denied nocturnal symptoms and could walk on a treadmill for 10 minutes, 3 times per week. Her FEV_1 continued to be stable at 75% predicted. When the prednisone was slowly tapered and discontinued over several weeks, she continued to do well.

Management of Acute Exacerbations of Asthma

The most effective strategy in the management of severe asthma exacerbations is prevention—early recognition of symptoms and signs of worsening dis-

Table 4.5 Classifying the Severity of Asthma Exacerbations

Symptoms, Signs, and Functional Assessment	Mild	Moderate	Severe	Impending Respiratory Arrest
Symptoms				
Breathlessness	While walking Can lie down	While talking Prefers sitting	While at rest Sits upright	
Talks in:	Sentences	Phrases	Words	
Alertness	May be agitated	Usually agitated	Usually agitated	
Signs				
Respiratory rate	Increased	Increased	Often > 30 per min	
Use of accessory muscles	Usually not	Commonly	Usually	Paradoxical thoraco-abdominal movement
Wheeze	Moderate, often only end expiratory	Loud through-out exhala-tion	Usually loud, throughout in-halation and exhalation	Absence of wheeze
Pulse per minute	< 100	100–200	> 120	Bradycardia
Pulsus paradoxus	Absent < 10 mm Hg	May be pre-sent 10–25 mm Hg	Often present > 25 mm Hg	Absence sug-gests respira-tory muscle fatigue
Functional assessment				
PEF percent pre-dicted or percent personal best	80%	~50%–80%	< 50%	
PaO_2 (on air) *and/or* PCO_2 SaO_2 percent (on air) or at sea level	Normal < 42 mm Hg > 95%	> 60 mm Hg < 42 mm Hg 91%–95 %	< 60 mm Hg ≤ 42 mm Hg < 91%	Possible respi-ratory failure

PEF = peak expiratory flow.

ease–and an action plan for early, aggressive treatment (Table 4.5). Consequently, patients should have a written plan to initiate and guide self-management of their asthma exacerbation. The action plan is not a substitute for physician involvement but rather a method to ensure early intervention. The action plan should include indicators of worsening asthma as well as specific recommendations on the use of β_2-adrenergic–agonist rescue therapy, the early administration of systemic corticosteroids, and when to seek medical care. Communication between patient and physician about worsening of

Table 4.6 Dosage of Drugs for Control of Asthma Exacerbation

Medication	Form	Dosage
Inhaled short-acting β_2-agonist		
Albuterol	Nebulizer solution (5 mg/mL)	2.5–5.0 mg q 20 min for 3 doses, then 2.5–10 mg every 1–4 h as needed or 10–15 mg/h continuously
	MDI	4–8 puffs q 20 min up to 4 h, then q 1–4 h as needed
Metaproterenol	5% Nebulizer solution	0.3 mL q 20 min
	MDI	4–8 puffs q 20 min
Systemic β-agonist		0.3–0.5 mg q 20 min for 3 doses
Epinephrine	1:1000 (1 mg/mL) subcutaneous injection	
Terbutaline	1 mg/mL subcutaneous injection	0.25 mg q 20 min for 3 doses
Anticholinergics		
Ipatropium bromide	Nebulizer solution (0.25 mg/mL)	0.5 mg q 30 min for 3 doses, then q 2–4 h as needed
	MDI (18 µg/puff)	4–8 puffs as needed
Corticosteroids		
Prednisone		All: 120–180 mg/d in 3–4 divided
Methylprednisolone		doses for 48 h, then 60–80 mg/d
Prednisolone		until PEF reaches 70% of predicted or personal best

MDI = metered-dose inhaler; PEF = peak expiratory flow.

symptoms, deterioration in lung function by peak flow values, diminished responsiveness to inhaled β_2-adrenergic agonist, or a loss in duration of effect are important steps that require a change in the treatment of asthma.

Inhaled β_2-agonists are the initial rescue treatment of choice (*see* Fig. 4.1 and Table 4.6) and often provide a prompt relief of acute airflow obstruction. This step usually can be started at home by the patient. Further treatment depends on the response to initial inhaled short-acting bronchodilator and the severity of the asthma attack. For example, complete or partial response in symptoms and peak flow can often be managed further at home by increased use of inhaled corticosteroids or the initiation of oral corticosteroids. However, symptoms sometimes become progressively worse over a very short time, despite the use of a bronchodilator; these patients need to be seen by a physician. Many asthma attacks, especially with moderate-to-severe exacerbation, require systemic corticosteroids to suppress and reverse airway inflammation. Patients should be instructed how and when to initiate a "burst" of prednisone.

The management of asthma exacerbations in the emergency room is outlined in Figure 4.2. The initial assessment should and often can be done quickly; in many cases, treatment is begun while the evaluation is still in progress. Signs of pending respiratory failure (*see* History and Physical Examination) should alert the clinician to the essential need to start extremely aggressive treatment in the emergency room (i.e., systemic corticosteroids, inhaled β_2-agonists, and oxygen) and to consider intubation with assisted ventilation. Patients without impending respiratory failure but with a poor response to aggressive treatment with bronchodilator require hospitalization for observation and the initiation of systemic corticosteroids. Severely hypoxic patients and those with early respiratory failure or a history of respiratory failure should be observed in an intensive care unit. Moreover, some patients respond to treatment with bronchodilators but have a recurrent episode of bronchospasm hours later; if this history is noted, oral corticosteroids should be started with initial treatment.

REFERENCES

1. **National Heart, Lung, and Blood Institute.** Guidelines for the Diagnosis and Management of Asthma. Bethesda, MD: National Institutes of Health; 1997; NIH Publication No. 97-4051.

2. **Busse WW, Calhoun WJ, Sedgwick JC.** Mechanism of airway inflammation in asthma. Am Rev Respir Dir. 1993;147:520–4.

3. **Adams PF, Marano MA.** Current estimates from the National Health Interview Survey, 1994. Vital Health Stat. 1995;10:94.

4. **American Thoracic Society.** Lung function testing: selection of reference values and interpretive strategies. Am Rev Respir Dis. 1991;144:1202–18.

5. **Li JT, O'Connell EJ.** Clinical evaluation of asthma. Ann Allergy Asthma Immunol. 1996;76:1–13.

6. **Pauwels RA, Lofdahl CG, Postma DS, et al.** Effect of inhaled formorterol and budesonide on exacerbations of asthma: Formoterol and Corticosteroids Establishing Therapy (FACET) International Study Group. N Engl J Med. 1997;337:1405–11.

SUGGESTED READINGS

Busse WW, Reed CE. Asthma: definition and pathogenesis. In: Middleton E Jr, Reed CE, Ellis EF, et al., eds. Allergy: Principles and Practice. 4th ed. St. Louis: Mosby, 1993:1173.

Evans DJ, Taylor DA, Zetterstrom O, et al. A comparison of low-dose inhaled budesonide plus theophylline and high-dose inhaled budesonide for moderate asthma. N Engl J Med. 1997;337:1412–8.

Pearlman DS, Lemanske RF Jr. Asthma: principles of diagnosis and treatment. In: Bierman CW, Pearlman DS, Shapiro GG, Busse WW. Allergy, Asthma, and Immunology from Infancy to Adulthood. 3rd ed. Philadelphia: WB Saunders; 1996:484–97.

Chapter 5

Allergic Skin Disease

Ernest N. Charlesworth, MD

Several decades ago, the skin was considered to be little more than a simple barrier to dehydration, environmental toxins, and extrinsic bacteria; however, we now recognize that the skin is a complex immune organ that is fully integrated with the immune functions of the bone marrow, lymph nodes, liver, and spleen. Lymphocytes possess a surface glycoprotein, referred to as the *cutaneous lymphocyte-associate antigen*, which specifically binds to the skin. The Langerhans' cell is the primary antigen-processing cell in skin. These cells have been shown to traverse to regional lymph nodes in which they then have an opportunity to network with lymphocytes trafficking to and from the skin. This paints the picture of the skin as being a very dynamic immune organ that is totally integrated with the other immune effector cells of the body. Mast cells, basophils, and eosinophils are also active players in this orchestration of inflammatory events that are observed with allergic skin disease. These events are complex and ultimately result in the release of pro-inflammatory cytokines, chemokines, and products of arachidonic acids, resulting in a cascade of immune inflammatory events that is recognized as allergic skin disease. The skin is the largest organ of the body, and allergic skin disease may be mediated by IgE-linked events (as noted with atopic dermatitis), by histamine liberation from mast cells (as observed with many cases of urticaria), and by T-cell–mediated allergic skin disease (as exemplified by allergic contact dermatitis [ACD]). This discussion reviews these three aspects of allergic skin disease; however, the reader is reminded that the skin has many other manifestations of immune dysregulation, including immunobullous disease, connective tissue disease, and a plethora of cutaneous manifestations of immunodeficiency disorders, such as HIV infection.

Atopic Dermatitis as an Allergic Skin Disease

The term *atopy* generally refers to respiratory or cutaneous disorders that are associated with IgE production. The term atopy was first coined by Coca and Cooke in 1923 to describe an unusual or "strange" skin disorder that was clearly associated with a familial tendency for both hay fever and asthma. The word *atopy* is derived from the Greek word *atopos*, which means "strange." Later, Hill and Sulzberger used the term *atopic dermatitis* (AD) to describe the chronic pruritic skin condition associated with elevations in IgE antibodies. Patients with AD generally have much higher levels of total IgE than patients who have only allergic rhinitis or allergic asthma, and there appears to be a strong correlation between the total IgE and the severity of clinical disease.

In addition to the association of AD with an elevated serum IgE, there is compelling evidence that the eosinophil plays an important role in the pathogenesis of AD. Significant infiltration of eosinophil-derived cationic proteins has been demonstrated in both the skin and the serum of patients with AD. This intense staining for eosinophil-derived major basic protein in AD skin, with only patchy staining in non-AD skin, suggests that the eosinophil is specifically targeted to the lesions of AD. The products of eosinophils are pro-inflammatory, and this phlogistic potential plays a significant role in activating the neurosensory nerve endings of unmyelinated c-fibers, which are responsible for the perception of itch. It is the itch that is the major clinical hallmark of AD; hence, AD is accurately referred to as an itch that "rashes," rather than a rash that itches.

The orchestration of the phlogistic events that result in intense dermal itching in AD patients is controlled by the activation of Th2 CD4+ lymphocytes. Peripheral blood lymphocytes from AD patients have been shown to spontaneously release both IL (interleukin)-4 and IL-5. Additionally, both acute and chronic lesions of AD have lymphocytes that express mRNA for IL-4, IL-5, and various endothelial cell adhesion molecules. When the available data are taken as a whole, it is clear that AD shares with allergic respiratory disease a rather specific upregulation of the Th2 phenotype and a down-regulation of the Th1 phenotype (1).

Diagnostic Criteria for Atopic Dermatitis

Unlike many other skin diseases in which primary lesions (e.g., papule, pustule, vesicle) can be defined, AD has no primary skin lesion. The clinical presentation of skin lesions with AD is induced by constant scratching and excoriations. This intense pruritus is the result of a lowered itch threshold. Acute flares of AD show a diffuse redness that may develop fine papules and vesiculation with rubbing. Ultimately, constant rubbing and scratching result in an intensification of erythema and postinflammatory hyperpigmentation.

Frequently, AD begins during infancy and early childhood years. This infantile form of AD usually involves the extensor surfaces of the extremities, face, trunk, and neck. Later, as the disease progresses into adulthood, it shows a predilection for the flexural aspects of the antecubital and popliteal fossae. With the progression into adulthood, the peculiar propensity for itching persists, and patients frequently develop a chronic hand eczema, which may be aggravated by occupations that require frequent wet or frictional hand work .

There are no laboratory tests that aid in the diagnosis of AD. The diagnosis of AD ultimately depends on a constellation of features, some of which are major features of the disease and others are more minor.

The criteria for diagnosis should include at least three major signs and symptoms listed in Box 5.1, allowing three or more of the minor features (also listed in Box 5.1) to be substituted for one of the major features. Because pruritus is the one unifying symptom for all patients with AD, if the patient does

---

Box 5.1 Major and Minor Characteristics of Atopic Dermatitis

Major characteristics

Pruritus

Early age of onset

Typical morphology and distribution

Flexural lichenification (thickening of the skin) and linearity in adults

Facial and extensor involvement in infants and young children

Chronic or chronically relapsing dermatitis

Personal or family history of atopy (e.g., asthma, allergic rhinoconjunctivitis, atopic dermatitis)

Minor characteristics

Xerosis (dry skin)

Ichthyosis, palmar hyperlinearity, keratosis pilaris

Positive prick skin tests to aeroallergens, dust mite, animal dander, and foods

Hand or foot dermatitis

Cheilitis

Nipple eczema

Susceptibility to cutaneous infection (especially Staphylococcus aureus *and herpes simplex)*

Perifollicular accentuation

Impaired cell-mediated immunity

not have a pruritic dermatitis, then a diagnosis of AD is unlikely to be correct. In fact, there are many diseases that may result in an eczematous dermatitis, including metabolic disorders, neoplastic syndromes, several diseases of immunodeficiencies, and chronic eczematous dermatosis secondary to ACD, psoriasis, and seborrheic dermatitis. In adults with a recent onset of a pruritic eczematous dermatitis, one should consider a broad differential diagnosis, including lymphoma, Sézary syndrome, ACD, and metabolic abnormalities (e.g., chronic renal failure) (Box 5.2). New-onset adult AD usually occurs in the setting of demonstrable atopy, with elevated total IgE and positive skin tests or positive radioallergosorbent tests to aeroallergens. The evaluation of the new-onset older patient with an AD-like eruption should include a complete physical examination (with attention to lymph nodes, liver, and spleen), complete blood count, electrolytes, liver function tests, and skin biopsy.

Immune Abnormalities

The concept that AD has an immunologic basis is suggested by the observation that patients with primary T-cell immunodeficiency disorders associated

---

Box 5.2 Differential Diagnoses of Acquired Adult Pruritic Eczematous Dermatitis

Lymphoma
Paraneoplastic syndromes
Sézary syndrome
Hypereosinophilic syndrome
Allergic contact dermatitis
Photo-induced dermatitis
    Systemic lupus erythematosus
    Subacute cutaneous lupus erythematosus
    Polymorphic light eruption
    Drug-induced phototoxic eruption
    Drug-induced photoallergic eruption
Drug-induced allergy
Metabolic abnormalities
    Chronic renal failure
    Hypercalcemia
Late-onset atopic dermatitis

with elevated serum IgE frequently have an eczematous dermatitis similar to AD. Wiskott–Aldrich syndrome is an X-linked, recessive disorder that has a pruritic eczematous dermatitis identical to AD, with the exception of the presence of petechiae resulting from an associated thrombocytopenia. Children with Wiskott–Aldrich syndrome have elevated IgE and IgA but a decrease in IgM. Patients with hyper-IgE syndrome present with the early onset of severe pyogenic skin infections of *Staphylococcus aureus* and an AD-like dermatitis in addition to coarse facies, growth retardation, and hyperkeratotic fingernails. Further evidence that AD is immune mediated is supported by the fact that nonatopic recipients receiving bone marrow transplants from atopic donors develop atopic symptoms, including AD, after successful engraftment.

Herpes simplex infection can be particularly severe and may be associated with an explosive dissemination, with generalized vesicopustules (referred to as *Kaposi's herpetiform eruption*). This is accompanied by a high fever, constitutional symptoms, and a 20% mortality rate. For many years, dermatologists have observed that empirical antibiotic treatment of AD patients frequently results in clinical improvement, even in the absence of clinical impetigo or pyoderma. The presence of *S. aureus* has been observed on the skin of 90% of AD patients but on the skin of only 5% of healthy patients. Despite the obvious colonization of the skin of AD patients with *S. aureus*, it is unusual for patients to develop actual invasive cellulitis, and the presence of invasive *S. aureus* should alert the clinician to the possibility of hyper-IgE syndrome or a deficiency of leukocyte adhesion (CD18). Boguniewicz and colleagues (2) showed that *S. aureus* organisms produce exotoxins (acting as superantigens) that may activate lymphocytes to produce pro-inflammatory cytokines.

Triggers for Atopic Dermatitis

The symptoms of AD are triggered by a plethora of potential aggravants, both allergic and nonallergic. During the warm summer months, occupational exposure to heat and increased humidity may result in a sweat-retention dermatitis (miliaria rubra and miliaria pustulosa) that provokes intense itching. During the winter months, increased skin dryness may be a significant contributor to intractable itching. Occupational factors may play a major role in the perpetuation and progression of AD, and career counseling may have a profound impact on young adults with AD. Exposure to strong industrial irritants and harsh environmental conditions has the potential to contribute to an inextricable escalation of symptoms, which can result in workplace disability. Because of the increased exposure of AD patients to topical creams and chemicals, the possibility of developing ACD far exceeds the theoretical decrease in the ability of CD8+ T lymphocytes to become sensitized. The resultant intractable itching contributes to continued scratching, creating a vicious itch–scratch cycle.

An appreciation of the potential role of inhalant allergens in the course of AD has been emerging. Much of the evidence has been anecdotal; however, Tuft (2a) reported a series of 136 patients with AD in which 121 had positive skin tests to ragweed. Of these patients, 64 had seasonal hay fever, asthma, or both associated with skin disease, and 13 had seasonal AD. Two of Tuft's patients were then challenged intranasally with ragweed, which was followed by an exacerbation of their pre-existing skin disease. In addition to exposure to seasonal aeroallergens, exposure to dust mite, animal dander, or both may play a major role in the disease pathogenesis of AD. This exposure can occur 1) by the direct contact between the allergen and the skin and 2) by absorption of antigen through the respiratory tract and the subsequent activation of skin mast cells distant to the portal of entry through the nose or lungs. Foods are also possible triggers in some patients with AD, although this may be of greater significance in childhood AD. In double-blind placebo-controlled studies of children in whom food triggers AD, egg, milk, peanuts, soybean, and wheat appear to be the most common culprits (3). In adults, foods are probably not a major trigger for AD, but certain foods should be considered if so directed by the patient's medical history; prick skin testing to these foods may be helpful.

Many children with AD will "outgrow" their eczematous dermatitis; however, severe AD extending into adolescence usually portends rather severe AD throughout adulthood. The triggers may change (e.g., children tend to lose food allergies), and adults in occupations with exposure to irritants or chemicals may have particularly recalcitrant disease. It is advisable, therefore, that career guidance during adolescence may be very helpful in minimizing future disease severity in young adults.

Treatment of Atopic Dermatitis

Because AD does not lend itself to "cookbook" treatment plans that fail to address the unique problems of the individual, the "art" of medicine and the clinical skills of the physician play a major role in the treatment of this disease. The triggers contributing to the flares of AD are many, and attention should be focused on controlling the trigger factors specific to the individual patient. Several years ago, the American Academy of Dermatology recognized the need to formulate guidelines for treatment of AD that focused on addressing the numerous trigger factors (4). Recently, the Joint Task Force on Practice Parameters (representing the American Academy of Allergy, Asthma, and Immunology; the American College of Allergy, Asthma, and Immunology; and the Joint Council of Allergy, Asthma, and Immunology) published a rather comprehensive and practical guide for the treatment of AD (5).

Recommendations for environmental modifications should include temperature and humidity control to avoid problems related to heat, humidity, and perspiration. During the summer months, air-conditioning tends to help maintain the temperature within the patient's comfort zone while removing excess humidity. During the winter months, an area humidifier may assist in increasing the relative humidity to prevent excessively dry skin. Skin infections (particularly *S. aureus* or herpes simplex) may be a recurrent problem requiring specific treatment.

Unlike allergic rhinitis and extrinsic asthma, immunotherapy has no proven place in the treatment of AD. There are anecdotal reports of exacerbation of disease activity and other reports that suggest improvement. Thus far, there are no good controlled studies that document a role for immunotherapy with this disease, and the use of this form of treatment should be considered experimental.

Corticosteroids (in conjunction with emollients to help promote hydration of the epidermis) are the mainstay of treatment (Table 5.1). There have been many positive advances in the pharmacology of topical corticosteroids, but inappropriate use of these drugs presents a potential disadvantage. Potent fluorinated corticosteroids should be avoided on the face, genitalia, and intertriginous areas; a hydrocortisone preparation should be used instead. The ultra-high-potency corticosteroid preparations (class 1) have the potential to induce atrophy and telangiectasia with great facility, and they also have the potential for systemic suppression of the adrenal–pituitary axis. For this reason, the ultra-high-potency corticosteroid compounds should be used only for very short periods of time in areas that are lichenified but not easily treatable with mid-potency corticosteroids. The goal of treatment is to use emollients and low-potency corticosteroids for maintenance therapy and to use the mid- and high-potency corticosteroids for short periods of time to address clinical exacerbations. Corticosteroid gel preparations are usually in an alcohol base that is irritating to the skin, which in addition to promoting dryness, limits their use to the areas of the scalp and beard.

Most patients with AD have dry xerotic skin, which contributes to disease morbidity because of the presence of microfissures and cracks that serve as a portal of entry to skin pathogens. This problem may become exacerbated during the dry winter months, and tepid baths followed by the application of a hydrophilic cream may give the patient excellent symptomatic relief. Emollients are less expensive than corticosteroids and are superb for controlling the pruritus of atopic disease while maintaining a soft texture to the skin (which is important for cosmetic and esthetic reasons). Hydrophilic ointments can be obtained in varying degrees of viscosity, and some patients prefer a thicker

Table 5.1 Topical Corticosteroid Preparations: Potency* and Vehicles

Group	Generic Name	Brand Name	Vehicle
I	Clobetasol proprionate	Temovate 0.05%	Ointment, cream
	Halobetasol proprionate	Ultravate 0.05%	Ointment, cream
	Betamethasone diproprionate	Diprolene 0.05%	Ointment, cream
	Diflorasone diacetate	Psorcon 0.05%	Ointment
II	Amcinonide	Cyclocort 0.1%	Ointment
	Beta-methasone diproprionate	Diprosone 0.05%	Ointment
	Mometasone furoate	Elocon 0.1%	Ointment
	Halcinonide	Halog 0.1%	Cream
	Fluocinonide	Lidex 0.05%	Ointment, cream, gel, solution
	Beta-methasone diproprionate	Maxivate 0.05%	Ointment, cream
	Desoximetasone	Topicort 0.25%	Ointment, cream, gel
III	Fluticasone proprionate	Cutivate 0.005%	Ointment
	Amcinonide	Cyclocort 0.1%	Cream, lotion
	Betamethasone diproprionate	Diprosone 0.05%	Cream
	Halcinonide	Halog 0.1%	Ointment, cream, solution
	Beta-methasone diproprionate	Maxivate 0.05%	Lotion
	Beta-methasone valerate	Valisone 0.1%	Ointment
IV	Triamcinolone acetonide	Aristocort 0.1%	Ointment
	Mometasone furoate	Elocon 0.1%	Cream, lotion
	Triamcinolone acetonide	Kenalog 0.1%	Ointment, cream
	Fluocinolone acetonide	Synalar 0.025%	Ointment
V	Fluticasone proprionate	Cutivate 0.05%	Cream
	Triamcinolone acetonide	Kenalog 0.1%	Lotion
	Hydrocortisone butyrate	Locoid 0.1%	Ointment, cream, lotion
	Fluocinolone acetonide	Synalar 0.025%	Cream
	Beta-methasone valerate	Valisone 0.1%	Cream
	Hydrocortisone valerate	Westcort 0.2%	Ointment
VI	Desonide	DesOwen 0.05%	Ointment, cream, lotion
	Aclometasone diproprionate	Aclovate 0.05%	Ointment, cream
	Triamcinolone acetonide	Kenalog 0.025%	Cream lotion
	Fluocinolone acetonide	Synalar 0.01%	Cream, solution
	Desonide	Tridesilon 0.01%	Cream
	Beta-methasone valerate	Valisone 0.1%	Lotion
	Hydrocortisone	Hytone 2.5%	Ointment, cream, lotion
VII	Hydrocortisone	Hytone 0.1%	Ointment, cream, lotion
	Hydrocortisone	Nutracort 2.5%	Lotion
	Hydrocortisone	Nutracort 1.0%	Cream, lotion

* Representative steroids are listed in groups from I (super potent) through VII (least potent).

preparation than others might require. Emollients offer a particular advantage when applied immediately after bathing, because they maintain hydration of the epidermis.

There are a multitude of hydrophilic ointments and emollients that may be used by patients with AD. The selection should be individualized and based on both patient preference and cost. Some AD patients may have a sensitivity to specific ingredients, (e.g., lanolin, certain preservatives or fragrances), a factor that must be considered when selecting a particular hydrophilic agent for long-term use. Some emollients are extremely viscous (e.g., Eucerin cream), which may be an advantage in extremely dry skin. Other hydrophilic creams (e.g., Cetaphil, Vanicream, Neutrogena) are less viscous and are preferred by many patients. If cost is a great concern, solid vegetable shortening (e.g., Crisco) may also be used. In rural regions of the country, local feed and animal supply stores carry large, inexpensive containers of hydrophilic creams (e.g., Udder Cream and Bag Balm), which are used for the treatment of chronic chafing of the udders of dairy cows. If patients choose to use one of these "udder creams," care should be taken to avoid products containing methyl salicylate (e.g., Udder Ointment) or other irritating ingredients.

Occlusive ointments are sometimes not well tolerated because of interference with the function of the eccrine sweat ducts, and they may induce the development of a sweat-retention dermatitis. Thickened and lichenified plaques of AD and atopic hand dermatitis, however, may respond best to a topical steroid in an ointment base. Clearly, an ointment base for a steroid delivery tends to enhance transepidermal penetration of the topical steroid and may increase the chances for cutaneous side effects when applied to the skin.

Therapeutic baths and compresses can be very effective in soothing pruritic skin. Following a therapeutic bath, the patient should pat dry and immediately apply a hydrophilic ointment, either with or without a topical steroid. Coal tar preparations may offer an antipruritic effect on the skin and can be used as a cream (5% liquor carbonis detergens) or an ointment (2.5% liquor carbonis detergens). Colloidal oatmeal preparations have a smoothing antipruritic effect on the skin and may be quite effective in controlling the itch. Wet dressings or wraps may be used to treat acute exacerbations; they have the potential to promote transepidermal penetration of topical steroid preparations. However, both baths and wet dressings have the potential to promote drying and fissuring of the skin if not followed by topical emollient use.

Antihistamines block the H_1 receptors in the dermis and may tend to ameliorate histamine-induced pruritus; however, it should be noted that there are no controlled studies showing benefit for AD. Because pruritus is usually intensified at night, the use of the classical antihistamines, with their soporific side effects, may be advantageous. The nonsedating antihistamines may then be used when alertness is more critical (e.g., during the working day).

In select severe cases, systemic corticosteroids may be used for short periods to bring poorly controlled patients under better control. The dramatic clinical improvement with systemic corticosteroids may be associated with an equally dramatic rebound flare, which may result in patient demands for frequent bursts of corticosteroids, leading to a "steroid addiction." If one uses a short course of corticosteroids, then an intensified topical program should be instituted in conjunction with the taper of the systemic corticosteroids.

Phototherapy using either UVB or PUVA radiation has been shown to be quite effective in selected patients with AD. In rodents, both UVB and UVA radiation have demonstrated a suppressive effect on the release of cutaneous mast cell mediators. Additionally, phototherapy has been used to great advantage in other conditions associated with intense pruritus (e.g., pruritus secondary to cholestatic jaundice, chronic renal failure, and systemic mastocytosis). Nevertheless, long-term use of phototherapy is associated with increased risk of skin cancer, including melanoma, and should best be undertaken by a dermatologist familiar with both AD and phototherapy.

Systemic immunomodulating treatments may be the future "standard of care" for the control of AD, and there are active investigative trials currently underway to determine the potential for immunomodulating agents in the treatment of severe recalcitrant AD. At this point, however, the exact role of these agents can not be defined. Interferon-γ is approved for the treatment of chronic granulomatous disease, but there are ongoing studies that suggest it may have a place in the treatment of AD. It was originally hypothesized that interferon-γ might benefit AD by the down-regulation of Th2 cellular responses; however, this treatment does not appear to reduce spontaneous IgE production. Nevertheless, studies in severe AD have shown that interferon-γ does result in clinical improvement. The exact role and long-term safety remain to be defined, and large multicenter clinical trials are currently underway. Tacrolimus (FK 506) has been used effectively for primary immunosuppression in organ transplantation and appears to be well tolerated (6). The mechanisms of action are similar to cyclosporin A; however, the safety profile is much better. The fact that topical application of tacrolimus results in local immunosuppression has prompted studies that have shown a greater than 65% improvement in clinical scores when applied topically. In this recent study, tacrolimus ointment was proven to be effective with only local burning and stinging as potential side effects. There are ongoing studies that should better define the clinical role of immunomodulating drugs, both topically and systemically, in the treatment of AD. Overall, the future looks brighter today for the treatment of this distressing disease than since the advent of topical corticosteroid treatments over four decades ago.

Case 5.1

A 33-year-old white woman presented with a 2-year history of urticarial lesions that waxed and waned with no particular pattern. She complained of moderate pruritus but also said that the lesions occasionally burned and stung. She denied any correlation with foods or menses. She was on oral contraceptives and a combination of H_1 and H_2 antihistamines. She said she was in good general health but complained of arthralgias without signs of frank arthritis or constitutional symptoms.

Her physical examination was normal, with the exception of generalized urticarial lesions, some of which had been present for 24 to 36 hours and displayed a "nutmeg" stippling of pigmentation. Other urticarial lesions had a hint of central clearing with a dusky discoloration.

Laboratory evaluation revealed an elevated erythrocyte sedimentation rate (44 mm/h); antinuclear antibodies, double-stranded DNA, and anti-SS-A and anti-SS-B antibodies were not detected. Complementary studies were all within the normal range. A skin biopsy of a lesion that had been present for 18 to 20 hours revealed a perivascular neutrophilic inflammatory infiltrate that was concentrated perivascularly but also had extended into the vessel walls. The endothelial cells were swollen with the deposition of fibrin, which is characteristic of fibroid degeneration. The histopathologic diagnosis was leukocytoclastic vasculitis.

An overall diagnosis of urticarial vasculitis was made.

The presence of urticarial lesions that persist beyond 24 hours and are associated with petechial staining is characteristic. Approximately 75% of patients with urticarial vasculitis will have arthralgias, whereas only 50% will have frank arthritis. The differential diagnosis includes systemic lupus erythematosus; however, the negative tests for antinuclear antibodies, anti-DNA, and anti-SS-A and anti-SS-B antibodies effectively rule out this possibility. The fact that the patient has a normocomplementemic urticarial vasculitis puts the patient in a favorable prognostic group with little risk of systemic involvement.

Antihistamines may help control the pruritus but usually do not control the immune-complex–mediated inflammation or the disease course. Some patients may benefit from a brief course of systemic corticosteroids; however, the risk of long-term corticosteroid use is not justified for a condition with a favorable prognostic outcome. Several other treatments have been used (e.g., indomethacin, colchicine, dapsone, and hydroxychloroquine) and are worthy of consideration.

Urticaria as an Allergic Skin Disease

Diagnosis of Urticaria

The clinical recognition of the usual urticarial lesion is not difficult. It generally presents as a raised erythematous wheal associated with varying degrees of pruritus, ranging from mild itching to an intense and unrelenting itch that interferes with work and sleep. The lesions show a variable tendency to be transient, usually waxing and waning over hours, if not minutes. In acute urticaria, lesions of less than 2-hours' duration show only subcutaneous edema on biopsy. In urticarial lesions that are persistent for several hours, lymphocytes will collect perivascularly. There are some patients in whom the lesions may tend to persist for longer than 24 hours; these patients deserve special attention. There are two groups of patients who may present with *persistent urticaria* (i.e., urticaria in which the individual lesions persist in exactly the same location for more than 24 hours). One condition is urticarial vasculitis; the other is the group of patients described by Hide and colleagues (7) in which histologically there was a mixed polymorphous cellular perivascular infiltrate and the presence of an autoantibody directed against the high-affinity IgE receptor on basophils and mast cells. For this reason, it may be worthwhile for the clinician to regard urticaria as a symptom—much as a febrile response is a symptom that might be triggered by several disease states, ranging from an infectious disease to a malignancy. If the urticaria involves primarily the dermis, then circumscribed erythematous pruritic plaques of subcutaneous edema develop. These lesions are often fleeting, lasting a few minutes to several hours. In one half of the urticaria patients, involvement of the deeper subcutaneous tissues resulted in angioedema. When urticaria and angioedema coexist, this appears to define a subpopulation of urticaria patients who have a worse prognosis than the majority of urticaria patients, and it is this subgroup of patients that may suffer recurrent episodes lasting longer than 5 years (8). Urticaria can be effectively divided into several broad clinical syndromes that may have different histologic pictures following biopsy of lesional skin (Box 5.3). In addition to a complete history and physical examination, a 4-mm punch biopsy of the skin can be a very effective tool for sorting the etiology of urticaria and as a means by which to classify the urticaria.

Aside from the persistent urticaria associated with the autoimmune-associated urticaria and urticarial vasculitis, there are several dermatologic conditions that may have urticarial-like lesions as part of their clinical spectrum, including erythema multiforme, pruritic urticarial plaques and papules of pregnancy (PUPPP syndrome), bullous pemphigoid, dermatitis herpetiformis, and papular urticaria (9). Box 5.4 lists several dermatologic disorders that may have urticarial lesions as part of their clinical spectrum. If one considers urticarial lesions as a potential spectrum of clinical manifestations of several cutaneous diseases, then it is not surprising that urticarial plaques may be more prominent with erythema multiforme than the classic *targatoid* or *bulls-eye* lesions as traditionally taught. Women in the third trimester of pregnancy, particularly primigravidae, sometimes develop a markedly pruritic urticarial dermatitis that is characterized by polymorphic lesions ranging from urticarial lesions to the PUPPP syndrome. The astute internist should not dismiss the association of urticaria and a neoplastic monoclonal gammopathy (Schnitzler's syndrome).

Box 5.3 Histology of Urticaria: A Guide to Causation

Sparse perivascular lymphocytic infiltration

Classic urticaria

Raised erythematous plaques

Dynamic state of waxing and waning

Frequent annular or gyrate appearance

Etiology

Urticaria secondary to antigen (e.g., food, drug, infectious agent)

Idiopathic urticaria

Mixed polymorphous perivascular infiltration

May represent an associated autoimmune dysfunction

Lesions may persist for several hours rather than exhibit rapid waxing and waning

Not associated with petechiae or purpura

Tend to be rather recalcitrant to routine antihistamines

Skin biopsy shows a mixed cellular infiltrate

Neutrophils, eosinophils, basophils, and lymphocytes

Etiology

Autoimmune-associated urticaria

Antithyroid antibodies

IgG anti–high-affinity IgE receptor (mast cells and basophils)

IgG anti-IgE antibodies

Anti-idiotypic antibodies

Urticarial vasculitis

Lesions tend to persist beyond 23 hours

Neutrophilic vasculitis

Eosinophils may suggest a drug-induced leukocytoclastic vasculitis

Mild constitutional symptoms

Arthralgia (not arthritis) and myalgia (not myositis)

Relatively benign course

Connective tissue disease

Distinct from "benign" urticarial vasculitis

Systemic lupus erythematosus may have urticarial lesions as part of a broader spectrum of vasculitis

Urticarial plaques have palpable purpura

Hemorrhagic vesicular and bullous lesions

Box 5.4 Diseases with Urticaria-like Lesions

Erythema multiforme	Papular urticaria
Bullous pemphigoid	Pruritic urticarial plaques and papules of pregnancy
Dermatitis herpetiformis	Paraneoplastic syndromes

Urticaria and angioedema are both frustrating and relatively common, affecting approximately one fifth of the population. By definition, urticaria lasting less than 6 weeks is referred to as *acute*. It is in this population that one is most likely to identify a specific cause or trigger. The two most common causes for acute urticaria are drugs and infections. We live in a time of "polypharmacy" in which many patients are on numerous medications (both prescribed and over-the-counter) and "natural" products. It may take quite a medical sleuth to sort out the ingested culprit from the chemical morass we introduce to our alimentary tracts. Foods that result in urticaria usually are related temporally to the ingestion of that particular food. If a food results in urticaria, urticaria should manifest within 30 to 90 minutes following the ingestion of that particular food, and it may be associated with other symptoms of an IgE-mediated reaction, such as abdominal cramping, diarrhea, nausea, or even bronchospasm, nasal congestion, or vascular instability.

Urticaria persisting for 6 weeks or longer is referred to as *chronic* and is perhaps the most vexing clinical challenge facing the physician. Most patients with chronic urticaria (and many of their physicians) believe that there must be a cryptic antigen that has thus far eluded detection, and they go from one physician to another looking for that extraordinary physician who will be able to identify the "allergy," eliminate the culprit, and restore their lives to order.

The etiology of chronic urticaria is generally not a specific allergen and is probably secondary to a decrease in mast cell releasability. This decrease in mast cell releasability may be the result of certain local cytokine production (e.g., RANTES) in the immediate microenvironment. The cause of acute urticaria is more likely to be discovered than the cause of chronic urticaria. Common causes of acute urticaria include drugs, food, and infections. The most common infections are viral. Viral syndromes may result in acute urticaria, sometimes presenting even after the viral symptoms have abated. A useful approach to causes is outlined in Box 5.5.

Angioedema Without Urticaria

Angioedema in the absence of clinical lesions of urticaria broadens the differential diagnosis to include both acquired and hereditary angioedema.

Box 5.5 Causes of Urticaria and Angioedema

Idiopathic
  Increased mast cell releasability
  Cytokine production on dermal microenvironment
IgE-dependent
  Atopic diathesis
  Specific antigen sensitivity (e.g., foods, drugs, therapeutic agents, aero-
    allergens, animal danders, Hymenoptera venom, helminths)
  Physical
  Contact
Complement-mediated
  Hereditary angioedema
  Acquired angioedema with malignant disorders or autoantibody
  Necrotizing venulities
  Serum sickness
  Reactions to blood products
Direct mast cell–releasing agents
  Opiates
  Antibiotics
  Curare, D-tubocurarine
  Radiocontrast media
Agents that alter arachidonic acid metabolism
  Aspirin
  Nonsteroidal anti-inflammatory agents

Hereditary angioedema (HAE) is an autosomal-dominant condition in which affected individuals have recurrent bouts of angioedema (without urticaria), which has the potential to be massive enough to compromise the airway. The gastrointestinal tract may also be a target of HAE in which patients develop abdominal pain, vomiting, and self-limited partial intestinal obstruction. HAE is due to an inherited C1-esterase–inhibitor deficiency, because of either a quantitative decrease in production or a dysfunctional protein. In the absence of C1-esterase inhibitor, C1 spontaneously becomes an active enzyme, cleaving and then inactivating C4 and sometimes C2. Most patients, therefore, will have a low C4, with C2 decreasing during acute episodes. Other forms of this angioedema have been described in which antibody to C1-esterase inhibitor develops as part of a paraneoplastic syndrome.

Management of Urticaria

The first priority in treatment of urticaria is the elimination of the causative agent, stimulus, or antigen; however, this is much easier said than done. For the majority of chronic urticaria patients, symptomatic treatment with classic H_1 antihistamines is the mainstay of management for their disease. The success of the classic antihistamines is somewhat limited by undesirable side effects, such as daytime sedation and anticholinergic-induced dry mouth. Because it is well documented that skin mast cells are triggered by unknown stimuli to release preformed mediators (primarily histamine and tryptase), it is only logical that antihistamines function best when taken as a prophylactic measure rather than just at the time of a flare of urticaria. Until the recent introduction of the newer low- and non-sedating antihistamines, physicians were reluctant to prescribe antihistamines for chronic daytime use.

Terfenadine, the first of the new generation of H_1 antagonists, was associated with a polymorphic ventricular tachycardia with prolongation of the QT intervals (*torsades de pointes*) and is no longer available. These problems have been eliminated with the use of fexofenadine, the metabolic metabolite of terfenadine. Astemizole also lacks the anticholinergic and soporific side effects of the classic antihistamines and has a slow onset of binding to H_1 receptors. Once bound to the receptor, astemizole then has an equally slow dissociation—an ideal characteristic for once-a-day dosing. Astemizole does result in an increased appetite in 3.2% of individuals taking the drug; however, its efficacy in the treatment of urticaria is well established. Loratadine, another of the newer nonsedating antihistamines currently on the market in the United States, is also more effective than placebo in treating urticaria. Its kinetics allow for once-a-day dosing because it is effective within a few hours of oral administration, lasting 12 to 48 hours following a single dose. Cetirizine, the carboxyl acid metabolite of hydroxyzine, is classed as a low-sedating antihistamine and has been shown to significantly reduce the incidence of erythema, wheals, and pruritus in both spontaneous urticaria and provoked urticaria in double-blind cross-over trials. Several investigators have demonstrated a decrease in the influx of eosinophils to the site of the antigen-induced, cutaneous, late-phase response following treatment with cetirizine (9). This anti-inflammatory property, combined with its excellent H_1-receptor blockade, is unique to cetirizine and may offer certain benefits in patients in whom the histologic picture demonstrates a mixed cellular inflammatory infiltrate.

Tricyclic antidepressants, such as doxepin, possess potent H_1-receptor blockade properties that are several orders of magnitude greater than that observed with the classic antihistamines. Because doxepin has significant soporific side effects, it is probably best used as an evening medication.

Although little evidence exists that H_2 blockers alone have any therapeutic effect in the treatment of chronic urticaria, there are some studies that support the effectiveness of a combination of H_1- and H_2-blocking antihistamines (e.g., hydroxyzine and cimetidine, respectively) in selected instances of urticaria.

Although antihistamines can control the symptoms of urticaria in many patients, the symptoms in some patients are so severe as to require glucocorticosteroids. Before committing a patient to frequent courses or alternate-day doses of glucocorticosteroids, a skin biopsy would better classify the urticaria histologically. Because prolonged use of glucocorticosteroids is associated with many side effects, some of the alternative drugs now being studied might offer relief from steroid requirements. Stanozolol, sulfasalazine, methotrexate (in urticarial vasculitis), colchicine, dapsone, indomethacin, and hydroxychloroquine have all been reported in the literature as showing some promise to reduce the amount and frequency of steroid need. For severe, unremitting, chronic urticaria, plasmapheresis might be used to remove possible aggravating circulatory serum factors.

Urticaria is a frustrating problem for both physician and patient. This problem is best approached by considering urticaria as a symptom of a much larger clinical disease spectrum. The clinical physical examination and the medical history remain as the two most important aspects of diagnostic evaluation for the clinician, with the laboratory work-up being directed by their findings. In the majority of patients, chronic urticaria is a self-limiting process, usually of unknown etiology. Factors that suggest urticaria is a benign condition without serious significance include the following:

1. A history of recurrent episodes over a number of years
2. The duration of the current episode for 3 months or more without other medical findings
3. The presence of dermatographia
4. Generally, a younger individual

The occurrence of the first episode of urticaria in a person over 50 years of age does raise suspicions regarding a specific etiology.

Frequently overlooked as a diagnostic tool, the punch biopsy is a valuable aid in sorting out the pathophysiology of urticaria, because the histopathologic findings can guide the physician in determining whether the process is most likely to respond to routine H_1 antihistamines or requires a more aggressive use of drugs (e.g., dapsone, glucocorticosteroids, or other steroid-sparing drugs) as the most appropriate treatment regimen. There appears to be a subgroup of chronic urticaria in which the patients seem to have an autoimmune disorder that results in the formation of autoantibodies directed against the thyroid or even against the IgE receptor on mast cells and basophils. Urticaria, its causes and cures, remains a slowly resolving puzzle for clinicians and patients alike.

Allergic Contact Dermatitis
as an Allergic Skin Disease

Previously both AD and urticaria were discussed as rather immediate types of allergic skin disease. The following discussion focuses on ACD, which is not an immediate reaction to an external allergen but rather a delayed reaction mediated by sensitized CD8+ lymphocytes and their cytokine effector products (i.e., Gell and Coombs, Type IV reaction).

When the skin is exposed to a potential external sensitizer, the Langerhans' cell processes the antigen and then presents the processed antigenic protein to complete the cell-mediated sensitization. The observed cutaneous lesions are confined to the general anatomical distribution of exposure, and the areas having the earliest and highest concentration of antigen exposure are the first to manifest clinical lesions, followed by several days of continual reactions in areas that are less exposed to the topical allergen. The lesions of ACD consist of raised erythematous plaques that have a tendency to develop vesicles and to display rather bizarre linear streaks (e.g., poison ivy dermatitis). The anatomic distribution can be helpful in providing clues to the clinician for identifying the potential allergenic culprit. This distribution may suggest an ACD to a topical cream, a chemical used in the workplace, or an outdoor plant, such as *Rhus* oleoresins from poison ivy, poison sumac, and poison oak (10).

Frequently, a cutaneous contact dermatitis may not have been an actual allergic reaction but rather triggered as an irritant reaction (11). In fact, as many as 80% of contact dermatitis reactions usually occur within hours of contact with the skin, resolving rapidly on removal of the offending agent. Additionally, the irritant reaction will frequently display a sharp line of demarcation between the involved and the uninvolved skin. As discussed previously, the patient with AD has a lowered threshold to respond to irritants and an increased opportunity to come in contact with potential contact sensitizers. A diagnosis of ACD should be entertained in all patients with the following:

1. Chronic hand eczema
2. Work-related dermatitis
3. Any chronic or subacute dermatitis
4. Chronic stasis dermatitis of the lower extremities

The differential diagnosis of ACD should include all eczematous skin disorders and some urticarial eruptions (e.g., contact urticaria). The location of the ACD will essentially dictate the differential diagnosis. For example, the differential diagnosis of a chronic hand eczema might include allergic contact dermatitis, irritant contact dermatitis, atopic dermatitis, pompholyx (dyshidrotic eczema), tinea manuum, and psoriasis.

Because the lesions of chronic ACD (as opposed to the acute lesions of ACD) may be nonspecific and eczematous lesions, the clinician should be familiar with a broader differential diagnosis of eczematous skin lesions, including cutaneous lymphoma, Sézary syndrome, psoriasis, parapsoriasis, photo-induced skin disease, and infectious diseases. A skin biopsy, when read by an appropriately trained dermatopathologist, may be quite helpful in ruling out disorders that may mimic ACD and in avoiding the unnecessary delay in the diagnosis of a cutaneous T-cell lymphoma or disseminated fungal infection in the immunocompromised host.

Latex Allergy

Latex allergy is becoming more recognized, manifesting either as an immediate hypersensitivity reaction or as an ACD to rubber accelerators and antioxidants. The primary sensitizing additives in natural latex ACD are the accelerators, which include thiurams, carbamates, and mercaptobenzothiazole (MBT). To shorten the lengthy vulcanization process to polymerize the natural rubber, accelerators are added as catalysts during the actual compounding. These chemicals help control the uniformity of the product and are important in providing the sulfur necessary for the cross-linking (vulcanization) of the polyisoprene chains. It is the thiurams that are the most sensitizing and may provoke an ACD in the wearer of latex gloves. Carbamates are also accelerators and are the second most common sensitizer, frequently cross-reacting in patients who are allergic to thiurams.

A combination of factors contribute to the potential for an individual to become allergic to latex. These factors include repeat exposure, frequent wet work with the hands, and the possibility of an increase in residual allergen coincident with the increased use of latex in the institution of universal precautions for exposure to blood-borne pathogens. This increased potential for exposure to latex allergens also increases the atopic person to the development of IgE specific to protein allergens, which may result in rhinorrhea, conjunctivitis, asthma, life-threatening anaphylaxis, and death. It is important to understand that natural rubber latex can cause two types of allergic reactions: ACD (mediated by sensitized T lymphocytes) and immediate hypersensitivity reaction (mediated by specific IgE antibodies).

Allergic contact dermatitis to latex gloves might present as a subacute or chronic pruritic eczematous hand dermatitis that would show a sharp line of demarcation between the involved and uninvolved skin. Patch testing with a standard tray (e.g., TRUE Test) might show positive reactions at 48 and 72 hours to black rubber mix, thiuram mix, and mercapto mix. The treatment of rubber or latex ACD consists of the avoidance of all latex-containing products and the substitution of vinyl gloves. Rubber and latex products are widely

---

Box 5.6 Latex Exposure in the Health Care Environment

Dental dams	Endotracheal tubes
Gastric tubes	Stethoscope tubing
Syringes	Tourniquets
Urinary leg bag	Resuscitation masks
Tidal breathing bags	Latex gloves
Suction catheters	Intravenous injection ports
Blood pressure cuff tubing	Hemodialysis components

---

used in modern society, and exposure can range from latex condoms to balloons to infant pacifiers. The medical uses for latex products are great, and exposure is almost unavoidable unless the clinician becomes acutely "sensitized" to the various routes of exposure (Box 5.6). Immediate hypersensitivity reactions to latex are potentially serious and are being recognized in more and more health care workers. Immediate IgE-mediated sensitivity is found much more commonly in women, patients who have undergone multiple surgical procedures, and individuals with spina bifida, intra-operative anaphylaxis, chronic hand eczema, an atopic genetic background, or a high risk of occupational exposure (e.g., health care workers and food handlers).

The IgE specific for the various natural proteins of latex also has the ability to cross-react with various food products (e.g., avocado, bananas, chestnuts, kiwi, and other foods) that are not phylogenetically related to one another, which suggests the presence of an antigen common to both the food and the *Hevea brasiliensis* plant (the rubber tree). Therefore, it is possible for a patient who has IgE directed against rubber latex to develop oral pruritus or even a more generalized syndrome after the ingestion of cross-reacting foods.

Case 5.2

A 25-year-old woman with a fair complexion and reddish-blonde hair presented with a 4-month history of a dermatitis involving the eyelids. The dermatitis was associated with marked pruritus. Her eyelids were puffy, erythematous, and appeared to be somewhat thickened (lichenified). There was no history of thyroid disease, proximal muscle weakness, or systemic lupus erythematosis. Her past medical history was unremarkable, except that she was intolerant to the use of diaphragms as a contraceptive device and was placed on birth control pills. The patient worked as an executive secretary and had no occupational chemical exposures. She used nail polish but did not wear artificial nails. She used a popular brand of facial cosmetics

Case 5.2 (continued)

that she was told was "hypoallergenic." Her eyelid makeup was applied using a sponge applicator. The makeup was removed at night with a nonsoap facial cleanser, followed by application of a nighttime moisturizer.

The patient was skin-patch tested using a commercial test (TRUE Test, Glaxo-Wellcome, Inc.). The patch tests were placed on the back and removed at 48 hours. The patient had a maximal reaction to mercapto mix, MBT, and black rubber mix.

An ACD to makeup sponge was diagnosed.

The patient has a typical history of eyelid ACD. The skin of the eyelids is very reactive, and ACD in this area may be secondary to chemicals used in artificial nails, nail polish, or both. Eyelid dermatitis may also be secondary to hair dye allergy even if the scalp itself is spared.

In this patient, the allergy is to the rubber accelerators that are used to speed up the rubber vulcanization process by cross-linking polymer chains. One would expect the patient to react to products containing latex rubber, including tennis shoes, insoles and adhesive shoe liners, latex gloves, rubber in undergarments, condoms, and other products. Nonrubber exposure to MBT may include certain cutting oils, antifreeze, anticorrosive agents, and veterinary products, such as flea and tick powders. Between 1% and 2% of individuals are sensitive to MBT, and this allergen is the most common cause of ACD from shoes.

Patch Testing for Allergic Contact Dermatitis

As alluded to in Case 5.2, there is one commercially available patch test kit, called the TRUE test (Box 5.7). It is simple to use and comes with an instruction video that demonstrates the proper application of the two preloaded allergens strips. Each strip contains 12 individual antigens and is left on the test site for 48 hours. It is then removed, and the cutaneous reaction is read based on a standard grading scale. The patient then returns 24 hours after removal for a second reading. If the patient is weakly reactive to a chemical at 48 hours and is negative at 72 hours, then the patient has an irritant reaction. If the reaction intensifies at the 72-hour reading, then an ACD may be indicated. Any clinician who does patch testing should be aware of the many potential cross-reacting agents, including the following:

1. Peruvian benzoin and balsam (which can cross-react with aloe vera)
2. Aniline dyes found in crayons (which can cross-react with para-aminobenzoic acid [PABA] in sunscreens)
3. Cashew nut oil in printer's ink or swizzle sticks (which can cross-react with poison ivy)

Box 5.7 Standard TRUE Test Allergens

Nickel sulfate	*p-tert*-Butylphenol
Wood alcohols	Paraben mix
Neomycin sulfate	Carba mix
Potassium dichromate	Black rubber mix
Caine mix	Cl+Me-isothiazolinone
Fragrance mix	Quaternium-15
Colophony	Mercaptobenzothiazole
Epoxy resin	*p*-Phenylenediamine
Quinoline mix	Formaldehyde
Balsam of Peru	Mercapto mix
Ethylenediamine dihydrochloride	Thimerosal
Cobalt dichloride	Thiuram mix

---

4. Pyrethrum powder (which can cross-react with ragweed, turpentine, or chrysanthemum)

Like dermatologists, general internists are trained to take a good medical history and correlate clinical symptoms with history and laboratory test results. When trying to unravel the mysteries of ACD, access to at least one of the several good reference textbooks is essential.

The definitive treatment of ACD is the proper identification of the allergenic culprit and subsequent avoidance of it. Unlike IgE-mediated immediate reactions to pollen, animal dander, or Hymenoptera venom, there is no effective immunotherapy available for delayed-type hypersensitivity reactions to contact allergens. It is important for patients to have a written list of the chemicals to which they are allergic and any other agents that might cross-react. Additionally, they should be instructed to read product labels to avoid exposure. The treatment of acute, widespread vesicular ACD may require the use of systemic corticosteroids tapered over 10 to 12 days to avoid a "rebound" flare resulting from an inadequate length of treatment. Pruritus may be controlled with the use of topical emollients and compresses containing colloidal oatmeal. Care should be taken to avoid the use of potentially sensitizing products that contain benzocaine or topical diphenhydramine (Benadryl), because these may complicate the clinical picture. Although total avoidance is the preferred treatment for ACD, the use of physicochemical barriers may offer some protection. Barrier creams are available for the *Rhus* oleoresins; however, they are of limited use for most contact allergens.

REFERENCES

1. **Cooper KD.** Atopic dermatitis: recent trends in pathogenesis and therapy. J Invest Dermatol. 1994;102:128–37.

2. **Boguniewicz M, Nicol HN, Leung DYM.** Atopic disease and the skin. In: Charlesworth EN, ed. Cutaneous Allergy. Cambridge, MA: Blackwell Science; 1997: 209–31.

2a. **Tuft L.** Importance of inhalant allergens in atopic dermatitis. J Invest Dermatol. 1949; 12:211–9.

3. **Sampson H, Scalon S.** Natural history of food hypersensitivity in children with atopic dermatitis. J Pediatr 1989;115:23–7.

4. **American Academy of Dermatology Task Force on Atopic Dermatitis.** Guidelines for Care for Atopic Dermatitis. J Am Acad Dermatol. 1992;26:485–8.

5. **Leung DYM, Hanifin JM, Charlesworth EN.** Disease management of atopic dermatitis: a practice parameter. Ann Allergy Asthma Immunol. 1997;79:197–211.

6. **Ruzicka T, Bieber T, Schopf E, et al.** A short-term trial of tacrolimus ointment for atopic dermatitis. N Engl J Med. 1997;337:816–21.

7. **Hide M, Francis DM, Gratton CEH, et al.** Autoantibodies against the high-affinity IgE receptor as a cause of histamine release in chronic urticaria. N Engl J Med. 1993;328:1599–1604.

8. **Charlesworth EN.** The spectrum of urticaria. Immunol Allergy Clin North Am. 1995;15:641–57.

9. **Charlesworth EN.** Urticaria and angioedema: a clinical spectrum. Ann Allergy Asthma Immunol. 1996;76:484–96.

10. **Beltrani VS, DeLeo V.** Allergic contact dermatitis. In: Charlesworth EN, ed. Cutaneous Allergy. Cambridge, MA: Blackwell Science; 1997.

11. **Marks JI, VA DeLeo.** Contact and Occupational Dermatology. St. Louis, MO: Mosby-Year Book; 1992.

SUGGESTED READINGS

Clark R, Adinoff A. The relationship between positive aeroallergen patch reactions and aeroallergen exacerbations of atopic dermatitis. Clin Immunol Immunopathol. 1989; 53(Suppl):S132–40.

Hanifin JM, Cooper KD. Atopy and AD. J Am Acad Dermatol. 1986;15:703-6.

Hanifin JM, Rajka G. Diagnostic features of AD. Acta Derm Venereol. 1980;92:44–7.

Jones SM, Sampson HA. The role of allergens in atopic dermatitis. In: Leung DYM, ed. Atopic Dermatitis: From Pathogenesis to Treatment. Austin, TX: RG Landes; 1996: 41–65.

Leung DYM, Rhodes AR, Geha RS, et al. Atopic Dermatitis (AD). In: Fitzpatrick TB, Eisen AZ, Wolff K, Freedberg IM, Austen KF, eds. Dermatology in General Medicine. 4th ed. New York: McGraw-Hill, 1993:1543–63.

Rietschel RL, JF Fowler. Fisher's Contact Dermatitis. 4th ed. Baltimore, MD: Williams & Wilkins; 1995.

Chapter 6

Anaphylaxis Including Stinging Insects

Robert E. Reisman, MD

Anaphylaxis is an acute allergic reaction, usually occurring within seconds to minutes after exposure to the causative agent, characterized by clinical symptoms that may include dermal, cardiovascular, respiratory, and gastrointestinal reactions. There are few, if any, parallels in clinical medicine where there can be such a dramatic and profound change from normal function and well-being to serious and even fatal pathologic condition. Although the pathogenesis of these reactions varies, the final pathway responsible for clinical symptoms is the effect of histamine released from granules in the mast cells and basophils and the effect of subsequent generation of other mediators, particularly leukotrienes and prostaglandins.

The clinical syndromes that accompany anaphylaxis are similar, regardless of the underlying etiology. The nature and severity of these symptoms are variable. People who have had recurrent anaphylaxis, such as from insect stings, tend to have similar clinical reactions each time. The similarity of recurrent anaphylactic reactions from other causes is not clear. To some extent, the amount of antigen exposure may be a factor, such as with individuals who react from allergen injections; higher doses may cause more severe reactions.

Risk factors for the development of anaphylaxis vary depending upon the underlying etiology. The presence of atopic disease (e.g., eczema, hay fever, and asthma) is generally associated with a higher incidence of anaphylaxis.

The most common symptoms of anaphylaxis involve the skin. These dermal reactions may vary from mild pruritus of the palms and soles to generalized urticaria, angioedema, and flushing. Cardiovascular symptoms include hypotension, shock, and if severe, loss of consciousness. Cardiac arrhythmias and myocardial infarction, possibly due to hypotension, have occurred during anaphylaxis. Respiratory symptoms may involve the upper or lower airway. Upper airway edema affecting the pharynx and larynx is one of the major causes of fatalities due to anaphylaxis. Asthma is another common reaction that usually occurs in individuals who have a previous history of asthma. Nausea, abdominal cramping, and diarrhea frequently accompany anaphylaxis. Rarely, uterine contractions have occurred, which may lead to spontaneous abortion (Box 6.1).

Symptoms of anaphylaxis usually occur within several minutes of exposure to the inciting substance. Less commonly, reactions have started 1 to 2 hours later. Biphasic reactions may occur with the initial symptoms, subsiding with or without treatment, followed by a recurrence of symptoms several hours later. It is presumed that these later symptoms are related to the generation and release of secondary mediators. This possibility has practical ramifications concerning medical treatment of anaphylaxis, as discussed below.

During the early phases of anaphylaxis, tryptase is also released along with histamine from the granules of mast cells and basophils (1). Serum tryptase levels rise, peaking at 1.0 to 1.5 hours and may remain elevated for a number of hours; thus, measurement of serum tryptase can be used to diagnose the occurrence of anaphylaxis. The best time to obtain serum tryptase levels is 1 to 2 hours after the onset of symptoms, but elevated levels may persist for 6 to

---

Box 6.1 Clinical Symptoms of Anaphylaxis

Dermal
    Urticaria, angioedema
    Flushing, pruritus
Respiratory
    Upper airway edema (larynx, pharynx)
    Asthma
Cardiovascular
    Tachycardia, cardiac arrhythmia, myocardial infarction
    Hypotension, shock, loss of consciousness
Gastrointestinal
    Nausea, vomiting
    Bowel spasm (cramps, diarrhea)
Genitourinary
    Uterine contractions

12 hours, depending upon the amount of tryptase released. Normal levels do not rule out anaphylaxis.

It is important to understand the pathogenesis of anaphylaxis in order to use diagnostic tests and provide subsequent prophylaxis or guidelines for future prevention. This approach is used in this discussion of anaphylaxis.

Clinical Syndromes

IgE-Mediated Reactions

Allergen- or antigen-specific IgE is the immunopathogenic mechanism responsible for most anaphylactic reactions, particularly those due to drugs, foods, and insect stings. Although present in the body in extremely small quantities, IgE is potentially very potent because of its ability to affix itself to the cell surfaces of mast cells and basophils. When two IgE molecules are bridged by an allergen, there is degranulation within the cells and subsequent release of potent mediators that are responsible for the acute allergic symptoms. This mechanism is also the one responsible for more common typical allergic reactions, such as rhinitis (hay fever), asthma, and urticaria.

In this model of anaphylaxis, prior exposure to the offending allergen is almost always necessary in order to stimulate the initial production of IgE antibody. Reactions following first exposure to a drug are uncommon. Reactions to first exposure to a food often can be explained by sensitization through breast-milk feeding. Approximately one third of individuals who have IgE-mediated anaphylaxis are atopic.

The overall incidence of anaphylaxis is difficult to determine and depends on the causative agent. For example, the incidence of insect sting allergy is estimated to be 0.4% to 3.0% of the population. Reactions to penicillin, primarily injectable penicillin, have been estimated to be 1 to 5 per 10,000 treatments. High-molecular-weight substances, such as horse serum, are highly sensitizing. Products derived from horse serum in the form of antipneumonoccal sera and diphtheria and tetanus antitoxin were commonly used years ago. Almost all patients who receive horse-serum products eventually develop IgE antibody and are at risk for the occurrence of anaphylaxis. Similarly, more recent experiences with chymopapain also suggest that patients can be safely treated only once because of its potent sensitizing properties.

The cause for anaphylaxis usually can be detected by measurement of allergen-specific IgE by the immediate direct skin test reaction or in the serum by an immunoassay. The direct skin test is quick, simple, and inexpensive. It causes a wheal-and-flare reaction due to the release of histamine resulting from the reaction of the allergen with IgE antibody fixed to the surface of mast cells in the skin, which is in a sense local anaphylaxis. Caution is advisable in highly sensitive individuals who could have a systemic reaction from even the very small amount of allergen used in the skin tests. There are several immunoassays that measure specific IgE present in the serum. As a rule, these tests are not as sensitive as the skin test, are more expensive, but are safer. These diagnostic tests can be used to verify or detect allergic sensitivity to foods, insect venoms, some antibiotics (e.g., penicillin), and a variety of other substances (e.g., latex).

During anaphylaxis, there is the possibility that IgE antibodies may be "neutralized" by the reaction with allergen. Following anaphylaxis, there usually is a rise in the titer of allergen-specific IgE, peaking in 2 to 4 weeks. For these reasons and also 1) to avoid a "refractory" period immediately after the reaction when diagnostic tests may be transiently negative or less reactive, and

Table 6.1 Classification of Anaphylaxis

Etiology	Pathogenesis	Diagnostic Test	Prophylaxis
Drugs	IgE antibody	Skin test	Avoidance
Foods		In vitro IgE antibody assay	Densensitization
Insect stings			Immunotherapy
Allergenic extracts			
Hormones			
Seminal fluid			
Latex			
Cold urticaria			
Radio contrast media	Complement activation (?)	None	Premedication with antihistamines, steroids, or ephedrine Hypo-osmolar contrast
Aspirin and NSAIDs	Leukotriene generation (?)	Aspirin challenge	Avoidance Densensitization
Exercise	Unknown (food allergy may be contributory)	None (food tests may be contributory)	Avoid food intake
Idiopathic	Unknown	None	Antihistamines, steroids
Transfusion (blood and blood products)	Anti-IgA (IgG or IgE)	Measurement of IgA	Washed, packed cells IgA-deficient gammaglobulin

NSAIDs = nonsteroidal anti-inflammatory drugs

2) to test at the time of potential maximum antibody response, the optimal time for skin or in vitro tests is 2 to 4 weeks after the anaphylactic reaction.

Avoidance of the offending allergen is obviously the most important recommendation for people who have had anaphylactic reactions. When this is not possible (e.g., in the case of insect sting anaphylaxis) or when not desirable (e.g., in the case of drug allergy and the need to administer that drug), "desensitization" procedures are possible. A number of protocols have been developed. The basic concepts involve administration of the drug or venom starting in very small doses and administering gradually increasing doses until the appropriate therapeutic dose has been reached. It is thought that this process leads to gradual neutralization of IgE antibody, which is responsible for the allergic reaction and stimulation of IgG antibody, which in turn may provide immunity or protection. Desensitization is not recommended for individuals who have food allergy. Although theoretically possible, early trials have been unsuccessful and have been associated with considerable morbidity.

The most common causes of IgE-mediated anaphylaxis are listed in Table 6.1. In the United States, the most common cause is the allergenic extracts used for immunotherapy. There are probably several million people who receive allergen injections. Recommended high-dose therapy is clinically more effective, but inevitably some systemic reactions will occur. Less common causes include insect stings, food, and drugs (e.g., penicillin). Several of these specific issues are addressed in more detail.

Stinging-Insect Allergy

Case 6.1

While mowing the lawn 2 weeks ago, a 40-year-old man was stung on the ankle by a yellow jacket. Within a few minutes, he became diaphoretic and developed generalized hives and pruritus. He complained of throat "constriction" and dyspnea. He was taken to the emergency room where he recovered quickly following treatment with epinephrine and antihistamines. Previous stings had been tolerated with no difficulty. His general health was good except for mild hypertension that has been controlled with propranolol for the past 2 years.

Case 6.1 describes a fairly typical scenario and a fairly common problem. Allergic reactions to insect stings constitute a major medical problem, causing about 40 recognized fatalities annually in the United States and being likely responsible for other unexplained sudden deaths. People at risk often are very anxious about future stings and modify their daily living patterns and lifestyles. Major advances in recent years have led to appreciation of the natural history of insect stinging allergy and appropriate diagnosis and treatment for people at risk for insect sting anaphylaxis. For the majority of affected people, this is a self-limited disease; for others, treatment results in a "permanent cure."

There are no reliable criteria that can predict or identify individuals who are initially at risk to develop insect-sting allergy. Stings prior to the one responsible for anaphylaxis usually have been tolerated with no adverse or unusual reactions. There is no relationship between the time interval between the previously tolerated sting and the subsequent sting that caused an allergic reaction. Systemic reactions have even occurred, primarily in children, after the first known sting exposure. Large local reactions, defined as extensive swelling from the sting site lasting from 2 to 7 days, are common but also do not predict future sting anaphylaxis. After subsequent re-stings, local reactions tend to recur, with less than a 5% incidence of anaphylaxis. On the other hand, the occurrence of many simultaneous stings (100–200) may sensitize people to venom, and anaphylaxis then may occur after a subsequent single sting.

Approximately 33% of people who have insect sting allergy are atopic, a slightly higher incidence than that in the general population. The majority of systemic reactions have occurred in people under the age of 20 years, with a male-to-female ratio of 2 to 1. This prevalence data may reflect exposure rather than any higher risk factors in younger people or men. Severe allergic reactions may occur at any age, although fatalities are more common in adults. The location of the sting may have some relevance. More reactions have been reported following stings around the head and neck, although reactions may occur following stings on any part of the body.

The clinical symptoms of insect sting anaphylaxis are similar to those occurring from other causes of anaphylaxis. Cutaneous reactions, urticaria, and angioedema occur in the large majority of individuals. In a Johns Hopkins University study (2) these were the only symptoms in 60% of children and in 15% of adults; severe symptoms may occur at any age. In our study of individuals who had potentially fatal anaphylaxis as defined by loss of consciousness, severe respiratory distress, or pharyngeal–laryngeal edema, there was a uniform age distribution (3). Thirty-three people (20%) were younger than 10 years of age, and 29 people (18%) were older than 50 years of age. Because the majority of insect sting reactions (usually of a mild-to-moderate intensity) occur in younger people, the relative incidence of severe reactions compared with total reactions is greater in adults. In the group of 40 people who had loss of consciousness, individuals were older and had a higher incidence of cardiac disease and β-blocker use. The majority of these individuals had no warning or indication of potential severe insect sting anaphylaxis. Twenty-five people had no previous sting reactions, nine had local reactions only, and six had previous systemic reactions (including one individual who had similar symptoms with loss of consciousness).

There are about 40 reported deaths per year from insect sting anaphylaxis. The majority of deaths occur in adults. The presence of cardiovascular disease, often found at autopsy, may explain the increased incidence of deaths in adults despite the higher incidence of anaphylaxis in younger people. Autopsy studies have shown a variety of pathologic conditions. Frequent findings include upper airway edema involving the pharynx, epiglottis, and larynx (which obstructs air flow); lower respiratory pathology with mucus plugs; pulmonary edema; and significant cardiovascular disease. On occasion, autopsy findings have been nonspecific, suggesting the possibility of an acute cardiac arrhythmia as the cause of death.

Insect sting fatalities are associated with an increased incidence of stings in the head and neck areas, the rapid onset of allergic symptoms, and minimal local swelling at the sting site (perhaps due to hypotension and the rapidity of the reaction). In the past, emergency medical therapy for treatment of anaphylaxis was rarely administered. In one study the records of 50 individuals who died of insect sting anaphylaxis and those of 100 individuals who had severe nonfatal anaphylaxis were analyzed (4). A major factor discriminating these two groups was the timely administration of epinephrine to the group with nonfatal anaphylaxis and the lack of epinephrine administration to the group who died (Table 6.2).

Anaphylactic symptoms usually occur within minutes after the insect sting. In general, the shorter the time interval is between the insect sting and the onset of symptoms, the greater the severity of the reaction. On occasion, reactions (primarily urticaria, rash, or angioedema) may start from 6 to 24 hours after the sting. Rarely, these delayed-onset reactions are also associated with more acute symptoms, such as throat edema and shortness of breath. Serum

Table 6.2 Suggested Effects of Epinephrine on the Outcome of Severe Insect Sting Anaphylaxis

Time Interval Between Sting and Epinephrine Administration (min)	Patients Receiving Ephedrine (%)	
	Nonfatal Outcome (n=100)	Fatal Outcome (n=50)
5–10	15	0
10–30	22	0
30–60	50	6
> 60	4	18
0	8	66
No data	1	10

Adapted from Barnard JH. Nonfatal results in third-degree anaphylaxis from Hymenoptera stings. J Allergy. 1970;45:92-6.

sickness–type reactions characterized by hives and arthralgias may occur from 7 to 14 days after an insect sting. These late-onset reactions, including serum sickness, are mediated by IgE antibodies. Individuals with these reactions are candidates for venom immunotherapy.

Studies of the natural history of insect sting allergy suggest that it is a self-limiting process for many people. The presumed effectiveness of treatment with insect whole-body extracts, which had been used for many years and is now recognized as impotent and lacking detectable venom components, can be explained only by spontaneous loss of allergic sensitivity. The results of intentional sting challenges and field stings in people who have had prior sting anaphylaxis and positive venom skin tests have shown only a 60% re-sting reaction rate. The occurrence of re-sting reactions is influenced by the nature of the initial allergic symptoms and age. The more severe the initial anaphylactic symptoms, the more likely there will be a re-sting reaction. For example, children with dermal symptoms have only a very benign prognosis with an exceedingly low (10%–20%) re-sting reaction rate. On the other hand, people who have had more serious anaphylaxis, such as loss of consciousness, have a very high re-sting reaction rate. In all categories of symptom severity, when re-sting reactions do occur, children are less likely to react than adults and symptoms tend to be similar to those that occurred during the initial anaphylactic reaction.

The occurrence or severity of the sting reaction is not related to the degree of skin test sensitivity or titer of serum-venom–specific IgE; thus, although IgE antibody is a prerequisite immunologic mediator of insect anaphylaxis, other undefined factors mediate the occurrence and severity of the clinical reaction. The medical treatment for anaphylaxis is the same as that for anaphylaxis due to any other cause. If the insect stinger remains in the skin, which most frequently occurs after honeybee stings, it should be gently flicked off. Care should be taken to avoid squeezing the sac, which could deposit more venom. Because the majority of venom is deposited quickly following the sting, this procedure may not be helpful unless done immediately after the sting.

People who are at risk for a systemic reaction from an insect sting should be referred to an allergist for evaluation. Therapeutic recommendations usually include insect avoidance education, epinephrine for self-administration, and consideration for venom immunotherapy. When outside, especially while gardening or in fields, individuals should wear slacks, long-sleeve shirts, and shoes. Cosmetics, perfumes, and hair sprays, all of which attract insects, should be avoided. Drab or dark clothing is more likely to attract insects. Particular care should be taken around food and garbage, which especially attracts yellow jackets. Individuals should be taught to self-administer epinephrine, which is available in preloaded syringes. They should carry epinephrine and antihistamines and use these medications at the first sign of an acute allergic reaction.

People who have had venom anaphylaxis and have positive venom skin tests are at risk for subsequent re-sting reactions and are candidates for venom immunotherapy. The selection process is influenced by age and the nature of the initial anaphylactic symptoms. Children who have dermal reactions only have a benign prognosis and do not usually require venom immunotherapy. All persons who have had severe symptoms should receive venom immunotherapy. Children and adults who have had moderate reactions are usually advised to receive venom immunotherapy, although this decision can be made on an individual basis.

Venom immunotherapy is highly effective, and subsequent reactions occur in only about 2% of treated individuals. Concepts are now evolving for duration of venom immunotherapy. Conversion to a negative venom skin test is an absolute criterion for discontinuing therapy. Three to five years of treatment appears to be adequate for most people. Individuals who have had severe anaphylaxis, such as loss of consciousness, and who retain positive skin tests may require longer treatment.

The individual described in Case 6.1 had no warning that he was allergic. A candidate for venom immunotherapy, he should receive information regarding insect avoidance and a prescription for epinephrine for self-administration. Allergy tests should be conducted to determine the specific venom to which he is allergic. The degree of skin test reactivity also provides the basis for the starting venom immunotherapy dose.

As noted, he was taking a β-blocker, propranolol. This class of drug potentiates any type of an allergic reaction, and individuals at risk for any types of anaphylaxis should avoid the use of β-blockers. Because he will be receiving venom immunotherapy, which carries a small risk of anaphylaxis, it is even more important that the propranolol be changed to a drug of another class.

Food Allergy

Perceptions concerning food allergy are extremely diverse, often confusing, and frequently based upon subjective interpretation; however, anaphylaxis due to specific IgE antibodies reacting with food protein is a serious and even fatal problem. Typical symptoms usually start within minutes of food ingestion. It is unlikely that symptoms occurring more than 2 hours after food ingestion are related to food allergy. The occurrence of food allergy may start at any age, but it is certainly more frequent in childhood. The most common offenders are fish, shellfish, nuts, peanuts (not a true nut), eggs, and milk. There are rare reports of anaphylaxis occurring from almost all foods, including poultry, grains, spices, vegetables, and fruits. Latex allergy, which is discussed later, occasionally is associated with food allergy, particularly tropical fruits such as banana and kiwi. Interestingly, some food allergies (e.g., nuts, peanuts, and fish) are lifelong. Egg and milk allergies, which are most common in early childhood, are self-limited and rarely continue beyond the age of 4 or 5. The intensity of the allergy may be exquisite. For example, reactions may occur due to exposure to small quantities of airborne food particles released during cooking, particularly in those with fish and bean allergies. Fatalities have occurred, especially following nut and peanut ingestion. Fruits, vegetables, and fish that have been processed and canned do not cause allergic reactions.

The diagnosis of food allergy is usually self-evident but when necessary can be confirmed by a carefully performed allergy puncture test or by measurement of serum-specific IgE. Treatment is directed at avoidance of food exposure. This can be difficult because there are often hidden sources of food exposure, particularly with nuts. People at risk must carefully read labels and constantly question restaurant personnel about details of food preparation. They should have epinephrine available at all times in case of a severe reaction. Allergy immunotherapy is not recommended at the present time for prophylactic treatment of food allergy.

Ingestion of fresh fruits and to a lesser extent fresh vegetables often causes itching, swelling, and irritation of the mouth and tongue, termed *oral allergy syndrome*. This reaction occurs almost exclusively in individuals who have symptoms of seasonal allergic rhinitis due to tree, grass, or ragweed pollens. The cause of the reaction often may be due to cross-reaction between allergens in food and pollen. As a rule, individuals with oral allergy syndrome rarely have more intensive symptoms such as anaphylaxis. Processed and cooked foods can be tolerated with no reaction.

Exercise-induced anaphylaxis is discussed later. For some individuals, exercise-induced anaphylaxis only occurs if food is eaten within a short period of time before exercising; within this group, specific food ingestion may be necessary. For example, some individuals require ingestion of a food such as carrot or celery and subsequent exercise to develop anaphylaxis. Suspect food etiologies can be confirmed by the immediate allergy-food skin test reaction. It is important to avoid ingestion of the suspect food or food in general for four hours before exercise.

Latex Allergy

Case 6.2

A 35-year-old emergency room female nurse presented with a 4-month history of sneezing, rhinorrhea, and nasal congestion with occasional cough. These symptoms

Case 6.2 (continued)

occurred only at work; she was unable to identify any specific cause. She had worked in the same job for 3 years with no obvious change in her environment or work duties. She took over-the-counter antihistamines with partial relief of symptoms. She took no medication on a regular basis. Her general health was good; however, she did have symptoms of seasonal allergic rhinitis when exposed to grass pollen.

When examined in the emergency room during a symptomatic period, she had bilateral conjunctivitis. Her nasal membranes were swollen and pale with watery secretions. Her lungs were clear, although she did cough during the exam. Subsequently, a prick skin test with latex solution was strongly positive.

It seems somewhat ironic that latex, which has come to symbolize safety in the public health response to AIDS, should itself become an occupational health hazard. Allergy to latex is now well recognized as a widespread problem in the health care community. Health care workers are most frequently exposed to latex in the form of gloves, but latex is also found in medical devices, such as infusion sets, endotracheal tubes, face masks, catheters, and tourniquets. Latex gloves are also used by hairdressers, food handlers, housekeepers, and law enforcement officials. More than 40,000 other products contain latex, including pacifiers, balloons, racquet handles, condoms, diaphragms, toys, and rubber bands. The latex allergen is readily adsorbed by the corn starch particles of powdered gloves. These particles become airborne and the latex allergen is thus readily inhaled.

Clinically, four types of reactions caused by latex product exposure have been described. The most common reaction is *contact dermatitis,* characterized by vesicles, erythema, and induration. This reaction is usually due to low-molecular-weight accelerators and antioxidants and can be confirmed by the typical patch test. *Contact urticaria* also may occur as a result of latex exposure. Airborne latex particles may lead to typical *allergic respiratory symptoms,* such as conjunctivitis, rhinitis, cough, and asthma. (The patient described in Case 6.2 was reacting to latex particles in the work environment.) The most severe latex reaction is *anaphylaxis.* Peri-operative anaphylaxis, often a difficult diagnosis, is frequently due to latex. It is imperative that allergic individuals be aware of their sensitivity. Most hospitals now have latex-free operating room environments.

Individuals who are frequently exposed to latex, such as health care workers, have a higher risk of developing allergy. A unique risk group is children with spina bifida or urogenital abnormalities, of whom one third to two thirds are affected. The intense and prolonged exposure to indwelling latex catheters is the main reason for this sensitization.

As noted previously, some individuals with latex allergy also may be allergic to exotic or tropical fruits, commonly banana, kiwi, chestnut, and avocado. The food allergy may either precede or follow the development of latex allergy, suggesting a cross-reacting allergen.

Diagnosis of latex allergy can be confirmed by an immediate skin test reaction. Unfortunately, there is at present no commercial latex preparation available in the United States for testing. As an alternative, latex-specific IgE can be detected by an in vitro test.

Individuals at risk must be educated to avoid exposure to latex products. In addition, for those individuals who have inhalant allergy, it is advisable to have medical, dental, or gynecologic examinations early in the day before the examining room may become "contaminated" with latex particles. Allergen immunotherapy is not a therapeutic option at the present time.

Allergen Immunotherapy

Allergenic extracts of pollens, molds, animal danders, and dust mites are commonly used for treatment of people with allergic rhinitis and asthma; this is known as allergen immunotherapy. Patients receive injections of substances to which they are allergic and which they normally encounter as airborne particles. Inhalation of allergens usually leads to upper airway and chest symptoms, rhinitis, and asthma. Injection of the same substance, which now leads to significant systemic absorption, can cause more serious allergic reactions. The incidence of anaphylaxis from allergen immunotherapy varies depending upon the sensitivity of the patient, type of allergen administered, dose of allergen administered, and dosing schedule. Nevertheless, most large studies suggest there may be as a high as a 5% to 15% incidence of anaphylaxis due to allergen immunotherapy. Generally, these reactions are mild and readily treatable; however, a small number of fatalities have occurred. Risk factors and appropriate guidelines for safe administration of allergen immunotherapy are discussed in Chapter 10.

Drug Anaphylaxis

Many drugs have caused anaphylaxis. The most common are antibiotics, chemotherapeutic agents, hormones, products made from heterologous sera, and products such as papain and ethylene oxide. Unfortunately, confirmatory diagnostic tests are only available for some of these drugs, such as penicillin, vancomycin, heterologous sera products, and hormones (e.g., insulin). When appropriate diagnostic skin test protocols are not available or have not been defined, carefully performed allergy skin tests with diluted suspect allergens can be performed. It is important that in these situations, appropriate control tests are performed using drug-nonallergic subjects.

Obviously, avoidance of drugs responsible for anaphylaxis is important. When administration of the drug is medically necessary, desensitization protocols usually result in tolerance to full therapeutic dosing. Attempted desensitization should be done only in carefully monitored and supervised situations, with available personnel and medication to treat anaphylaxis. Specific protocols are described in Chapter 7.

Cold Urticaria

Urticaria and angioedema may develop following exposure to cold temperatures, primarily on exposed areas. Once recognized, this problem is usually easily controlled by minimizing cold exposure and by using antihistamines, particularly cyproheptadine, when needed. Acute anaphylaxis may occur if there is sudden exposure of large body areas to relatively cold temperatures, such as in swimming pools or lakes.

The etiology of cold urticaria is unknown, although there are numerous anecdotal reports of symptoms starting after insect sting reactions. About half of people with cold urticaria have an IgE-type antibody demonstrable by the old passive transfer technique.

Non–IgE-Mediated Reactions

The chemical mediators that cause anaphylaxis may be released from mast cells and basophils by non–IgE-dependent mechanisms. The term *anaphylactoid* has been applied by some investigators to describe this event. The clinical syndrome, however, is different because the allergic symptoms depend on the mediator release, not the specific pathogenesis. Aspirin and radio contrast media are common examples of causes of these reactions (*see* Table 6.1).

Diagnostic immediate skin test reactions or measurement of serum antibody cannot be used for the diagnosis of non–IgE-mediated anaphylaxis. Desensitization procedures, except for aspirin and aspirin-like drugs, are not effective.

Exercise-Induced Anaphylaxis

Case 6.3

A 22-year-old woman developed generalized hives, lightheadedness, and shortness of breath while running. She had been jogging about 45 minutes when the symptoms started. She had jogged daily for several years and had noted mild pruritus in the groin, axilla, and palms on several other occasions. Her health is good. She does have mild summer-time hay fever.

This individual developed typical symptoms of anaphylaxis while exercising. This syndrome, which is now well defined, was first observed and described over 15 years ago, concomitant with the increased attention to physical fitness. The clinical symptoms are typical of anaphylaxis from any cause. There is often initial pruritus of the palms, soles, and groin, which may progress to the more serious symptoms of vascular collapse or upper airway obstruction. Symptoms are not easy to reproduce. Individuals may exercise to the same extent repeatedly and have a sporadic recurrence of symptoms. This observation suggests that there may be factors in addition to exercise that modulate this reaction. One identified factor for some individuals is food ingestion or even ingestion of a specific food within 4 to 6 hours before exercise. To date, the natural history of exercise anaphylaxis has not been well defined.

Awareness of this entity often will make the diagnosis of exercise-induced anaphylaxis possible. It is not unusual to obtain a history of recurrent anaphylaxis that the patient does not associate with exercise. Once the diagnosis is suspected, the issues of food ingestion and perhaps specific allergy food testing can be addressed.

Treatment is directed at prevention. Individuals with exercise-induced anaphylaxis should not exercise alone. Emergency medication should be available and administered at the first sign of a reaction. Food ingestion should be avoided for 4 to 6 hours before exercise. It is not known whether prophylactic antihistamine administration will prevent the occurrence of exercise-induced anaphylaxis. Certainly at the first sign of any type of allergic symptoms, exercise should be discontinued.

Exercise anaphylaxis should be differentiated from two other syndromes: exercise-induced asthma and cholinergic urticaria. Almost all patients with asthma can have exercise-induced exacerbations. Some people develop small hives as the result of excessive heat, frequently as the result of exercise. Neither of these syndromes is associated with multiple symptoms of generalized anaphylaxis and thus the distinction is usually readily made.

Contrast Media

Case 6.4

A 60-year-old man with angina is scheduled for coronary angiography. Five years ago he developed generalized hives and hypotension following injection of contrast media for an intravenous pyelogram. He has had no other known allergies. He has never had hives or allergic-like symptoms. Angiography is now strongly recommended to assess the degree of heart disease.

Case 6.4 presents another common scenario. It is estimated that allergic reactions due to the standard ionic hyperosmolar contrast media occur in 5% to 12% of patients with about 500 deaths reported annually. The underlying mechanism for these reactions has not been established, but complement activation (which subsequently leads to mediator release) has been suggested. There are no diagnostic tests that reliably identify individuals at risk for an allergic reaction due to contrast media. Because the condition is not IgE mediated, there are no allergy skin tests or in vitro tests available to detect potential reactions. Allergy to contrast media is unrelated to fish allergy, a common misconception. The presence of iodine in fish and contrast media is not a common antigenic factor. A trial administration of a small amount of contrast media does not detect potential reactions to the therapeutic dose.

The major risk factor for an allergic reaction from contrast media is a history of a prior reaction. It is estimated that between 40% and 60% of individuals who have had a previous reaction will react again following re-exposure. Other risk factors are the presence of asthma and the history of multiple allergies, such as drug and food reactions and rhinitis.

For individuals at potential risk for contrast media allergic reactions, there are two approaches: the use of prophylactic or preventive medication and the use of hypo-osmolar (nonionic) contrast media. The previous administration of antihistamines and steroids significantly reduces the risk of an allergic reaction from contrast media to about 5% to 10%. The addition of ephedrine may further reduce this reaction.

Some physicians also recommend the use of an H_2 blocking agent such as cimetidine. One commonly recommended and well-studied effective regimen is as follows:

1. Diphenhydramine, 50 mg, either orally or parentally 1 hour before the procedure.
2. Prednisone, 50 mg, in three doses approximately 1, 7, and 13 hours before the procedure. In addition, ephedrine, 25 mg, can be given 1 hour beforehand.

The second approach is to use hypo-osmolar, or nonionic, contrast media (5). The risk of reactions from these materials is low, estimated at approximately 0.4%. The routine use of hypo-osmolar contrast media for all patients obviously would be ideal but is limited by its cost, which is approximately 6 to 10 times that of the hyper-osmolar contrast media. This dilemma regarding routine use of a safer preparation does raise ethical and legal as well as medical issues.

Individuals at potential risk for reactions to contrast media, such as described in Case 6.4, should receive both prophylactic medication (steroids, antihistamines, and possibly ephedrine) and hypo-osmolar contrast media. The combination of this approach should reduce the potential risk of an allergic reaction to 1% to 2% or less.

Reactions from myelographic and arthrographic procedures are much less frequent than those following intravascular contrast administration. Nevertheless, individuals at potential risk for contrast media reactions who undergo these procedures should receive medical prophylaxis and nonionic radio contrast.

Blood Products

Anaphylaxis during blood or blood product administration is usually caused by the reaction of IgA in the transfused product with the recipients anti-IgA IgG or anti-IgA IgE. Approximately 1 in 600 individuals lack IgA. Exposure to IgA by transfusion or pregnancy may stimulate production of an anti-IGA IgG antibody or an anti-IgA IgE antibody. Subsequent exposure to IgA results in anaphylaxis, perhaps mediated by complement activation when IgG is involved. Recognition of this etiology is important, and subsequent transfusions with washed, packed cells can be administered without a reaction. The same mechanism may be responsible for anaphylaxis during intravenous gammaglobulin infusion. The use of a relatively IgA-deficient gammaglobulin preparations will avoid subsequent reactions.

During administration of intravenous gammaglobulin, clinical symptoms of fever, fatigue, and generalized aches may occur. Prophylaxis includes pretreatment with antihistamines and aspirin and slowing the rate of gammaglobulin infusion.

Aspirin and Other Nonsteroidal Anti-Inflammatory Drugs

Case 6.5

A 30-year-old woman has a 5-year history of progressive symptoms of nasal stuffiness associated with postnasal drainage, occasional rhinorrhea, and a feeling of "pressure" above and below the eyes. During the past year, her smell perception has been diminished, and she is now able to detect only very strong odors. These nasal symptoms are perennial and exacerbated by weather changes and exposure to airborne irritants such as smoke. Nasal secretions are described as watery and minimal. During the past 2 months, she has become aware of chest tightness and wheezing that occur during and following exercise. Antihistamine decongestant medications have been taken with no obvious benefit. She is a nonsmoker and is not exposed to smoke on a regular basis. Her general health is good.

Two weeks before presentation she took aspirin, 650 mg, because of headache. Within 5 minutes, she noticed increased shortness of breath associated with wheezing and chest constriction. She used an inhaled bronchodilator that had been prescribed for her husband's asthma and within a short time the symptoms resolved.

Pertinent physical examination findings were swollen, pale nasal membranes and small bilateral nasal polyps. The chest examination and peak flow were normal.

The individual described in Case 6.5 had an acute allergic-like reaction caused by aspirin ingestion. This clinical reaction to aspirin and other nonsteroidal anti-inflammatory drugs (NSAIDs) occurs in individuals who have a classic triad of nasal polyps, asthma, and aspirin sensitivity (aspirin triad or Samter's triad) (6). The age of onset is usually in late adolescence through mid 30s. There is a greater incidence in women than men. Initial symptoms are usually nasal, with rhinorrhea, congestion, and ultimately anosmia. Usually, although not always, asthma occurs after the onset of the nasal symptoms. Most individuals are not atopic, and standard allergy tests are usually negative. There is a fairly profound eosinophilia in nasal secretions and nasal polyps. Pansinusitis is frequent, and computed tomography scans show moderate-to-marked polypoid membrane swelling. Although the degree and extent of asthma may be variable, it is not unusual for asthma to be chronic and severe and require maintenance steroid therapy. The usual medical treatment includes the regular use of intranasal and inhaled steroids and the periodic use of oral steroids for exacerbations. When nasal and sinus symptoms are persistent and require frequent steroid therapy, endoscopic surgery is advisable.

Within a short period of time, 5 minutes to several hours after ingestion of aspirin or other NSAIDs drugs, there is a fairly typical clinical reaction characterized by acute and often severe asthma with associated nasal congestion and facial flush. Asthma may require repeated aerosol bronchodilator treatment as well as steroids, epinephrine, and oxygen if severe.

This type of reaction caused by aspirin should be distinguished from other allergic reactions. Aspirin or other NSAIDs may cause generalized urticaria and frequently exacerbate urticaria in individuals with chronic urticaria. In addition, typical anaphylaxis (described previously) also may occur following aspirin ingestion. In this situation, anaphylaxis is probably mediated by aspirin-specific IgE, and other NSAIDs might be tolerated without reaction.

The incidence of this respiratory type of aspirin reaction is between 9% and 31% of all asthmatics, between 30% and 40% of individuals who have rhinosinusitis and nasal polyps, and between 70% and 97% of individuals who have had previous aspirin-induced reactions.

The mechanism responsible for these respiratory reactions is related to the biochemical properties of aspirin and NSAIDs drugs. These drugs block the formation of prostaglandins and thromboxanes and shift the metabolism of arachidonic acid from the cyclooxygenase pathway to the lipoxygenase pathway, leading to the formation of leukotrienes. There are reports that leukotriene antagonists can prevent the occurrence of clinical reactions in aspirin-sensitive asthmatics. Because their biochemical function is similar, all NSAIDs may cause these reactions. Drugs that weakly inhibit the cyclo-oxygenase pathway, such as acetaminophen, are usually well tolerated; however, they may also cause reactions in higher doses.

Currently there is no available diagnostic test for detection of aspirin sensitivity. As a rule, the diagnosis is self-evident because the acute reaction usually occurs in the setting of a fairly typical clinical syndrome. For individuals who have never experienced an adverse reaction from aspirin and do have nasal polyps, sinusitis, and asthma, it is prudent to recommend avoidance of all NSAIDs because there is no way to predict when the initial reaction may occur or how severe it may be.

It may be desirable for patients with this syndrome to tolerate aspirin. Examples include individuals who have inflammatory arthritis and those who have cardiovascular disease for which anticoagulation is advisable. Recently, there also have been suggestions that the basic disease process, rhinitis, sinusitis, and asthma may improve if individuals are able to tolerate daily doses of aspirin. The possibility of administering aspirin without adverse reactions originates from several fortuitous observations that following aspirin challenges and induction of symptoms there is a refractory period during which aspirin is tolerated with no problem. Refined studies now have shown that this refractory period lasts from 2 to 5 days. As long as the aspirin administration is then maintained, no reaction will occur. These studies suggest that all aspirin-sensitive individuals who have this respiratory reaction are capable of being desensitized and that the desensitized state can be maintained indefinitely if aspirin is taken daily. Patients who have urticaria and angioedema due to aspirin are much more difficult, if not impossible, to desensitize.

The method of aspirin desensitization involves administration of small, gradually increasing doses of aspirin until the asthmatic reaction occurs. At this point, the symptoms are treated, which often requires intensive medication. The aspirin desensitization program is resumed the following day, usually with no difficulty. Once a full dose of aspirin is tolerated, it may be given daily. The desensitization state applies to all of the nonsteroidal anti-inflammatory drugs; thus, it is possible for those individuals (particularly those with arthritis) to tolerate medication with no difficulty. It is obviously very risky to attempt this procedure in individuals who have cardiovascular disease because the end point is asthma, which may not respond readily to treatment.

Idiopathic Anaphylaxis

Idiopathic anaphylaxis is defined as anaphylaxis that occurs without an identifiable cause. The diagnosis depends on the failure to find a specific cause for anaphylaxis despite an intensive search for the usual etiologies, such as foods, drugs, stings, bites, or exercise. The clinical syndrome is exactly the same as anaphylaxis from a defined cause. The overall incidence is low.

Idiopathic anaphylaxis has been classified depending on the frequency and severity of symptoms. This classification has been used as a guideline for prophylactic therapy. Individuals at risk are advised to keep medication available for treatment of anaphylaxis, which includes epinephrine, antihistamines, and steroids. These therapeutic principles are described in the next section.

It has been suggested that when episodes of idiopathic anaphylaxis occur six or more times a year, prophylactic medical therapy is indicated (7). Antihistamines are given daily. Initially, prednisone in fairly large doses (60–100 mg/d) is given for 7 to 14 days and then slowly decreased. If the antihistamine alone does not control recurrent episodes, alternate-day prednisone on a long-term basis may be necessary. Those patients who have more severe life-threatening anaphylactic symptoms usually require more steroid therapy.

Medical Treatment of Anaphylaxis

Anaphylaxis should be treated at the earliest indication of signs and symptoms. There should be rapid assessment of the two major, potentially life-threatening reactions: airway patency (particularly upper airway swelling) and cardiovascular function. Concomitantly, appropriate medication should be administered immediately.

The rapid assessment includes removal of the offending allergen if still present, measurement of vital signs (e.g., pulse and blood pressure), and assessment of airway patency. The initial medical treatment is the administration of 1:1000 epinephrine. The usual adult dose is 0.3 to 0.5 mg administered subcutaneously. Because epinephrine has a short half-life, this dose can be repeated every 10 to 15 minutes. If shock and hypotension are present, the epinephrine, diluted 1:10,000, can be administered slowly intravenously. Epinephrine should be administered even if the only presenting signs of anaphylaxis are hives or pruritus. Antihistamines may be helpful in relieving cutaneous symptoms such as hives and flushing. The usual recommended dose is diphenhydramine, 50 mg, intramuscularly or intravenously. There is some dispute about the effectiveness of H_2 antagonists, such as ranitidine or cimetidine. These medications may add additional benefit, particularly in improving the cardiovascular symptoms. The usual dose is ranitidine, 50 mg (intravenously or intramuscularly) or cimetidine, 200 to 300 mg (intravenously or intramuscularly).

The symptom complex will dictate other therapy. If there is cardiovascular or respiratory impairment, oxygen should be administered by face mask or nasal cannula. Asthma that is not responsive to epinephrine alone might be helped by aerosol bronchodilators.

Patients who are taking β-blocking agents may have more severe anaphylactic reactions and may not be as responsive to epinephrine. In this situation, the use of glucagon may be useful. The usual dose is 1 to 5 mg intravenously over 2 minutes, followed by an infusion of 5 to 15 µ/min. Hypotension may require the use of large amounts of intravenous fluid such as normal saline. Vasopressors may also be necessary to relieve hypotension if these other measures are not effective.

Steroid therapy is also recommended for moderate-to-severe anaphylaxis. Although the beneficial effect of steroids may take several hours, these medications are given in an effort to prevent late-onset reactions. Steroids should be given in large doses such as 300 to 400 mg of hydrocortisone or 60 to 80 mg of methylprednisolone intravenously immediately and repeated every 4 hours as needed. Large oral doses are also usually sufficient.

After an initial response to therapy, anaphylactic symptoms may recur several hours later. This is particularly true if the initial medication (e.g., epinephrine and antihistamines) has provided therapeutic benefit but has since been metabolized or eliminated from the body. If the anaphylaxis is severe, it is prudent to keep patients under observation for at least 4 to 6 hours to avoid recurrence after hospital or emergency room discharge. Even in the case of milder symptoms, many physicians advise the use of antihistamines (e.g., diphenhydramine, 50 mg, every 6 hours) and steroids (e.g., prednisone, 20 mg, every 6–8 hours) for 24 to 48 hours after amelioration of acute symptoms.

REFERENCES

1. **Schwartz LB, Yunginger JW, Miller J, et al.** The time course of appearance and disappearance of human mast cell tryptase in the circulation after anaphylaxis. J Clin Invest. 1989;83:1551–5.

2. **Golden DBK, Lichtenstein LM.** Insect sting allergy. In: Kaplan AP, ed. Allergy. New York: Churchill Livingstone; 1985:507.

3. **Lantner R, Reisman RE.** Clinical and immunologic features and subsequent course of patients with severe insect sting anaphylaxis. J Allergy Clin Immunol. 1989;94:900–6.

4. **Barnard JH.** Nonfatal results in third degree anaphylaxis from Hymenoptera stings. J Allergy. 1970;45:92–96.

5. **Greenberger P, Patterson R.** Beneficial effects of lower osmolality contrast media in pretreated high risk patients. J Allergy Clin Immunol. 1991;87:867–72.

6. **Samter M, Beers RF Jr.** Intolerance to aspirin. Ann Intern Med. 1968;68:975–83.

7. **Patterson R, Stoloff R, Greenberger DA, Grammer LC, Harris KE.** Algorithms for the diagnosis and management of idiopathic anaphylaxis. Ann Allergy. 1993;71:40–4.

SUGGESTED READINGS

General

Kemp SF, Lockey RF, Lieberman P, et al. Anaphylaxis: a review of 266 cases. Arch Int Med. 1995;155:1749–54.

Smith PL, Kagey-Sobotka A, Bleecker ER, et al. Physiologic manifestations of human anaphylaxis. J Clin Invest. 1980;66:1072–80.

Toogood JH. Beta-blocker therapy and the risk of anaphylaxis. Can Med Assoc J. 1987;136:929–33.

The use of epinephrine in the treatment of anaphylaxis (Position Paper). J Allergy Clin Immunol. 1994;94:666–8.

Winbery SL, Lieberman PL. Anaphylaxis. Immunol Allergy Clin North Am. 1995;15:447–75.

Stinging Insects

Golden DBK, Kwitervovich KA, Kagey-Sobotka A, et al. Discontinuing venom immunotherapy: outcome after five years. J Allergy Clin Immunol. 1996;97:479–87.

Reisman RE. Insect stings. N Engl J Med. 1994;331:523–7.

Valentine MD, Schuberth KC, Kagey-Sobtka A, et al. The value of immunotherapy with venom in children with allergy to insect stings. N Engl J Med. 1991;23:1601–3.

Food Allergy

Atkins FM, Steinberg SS, Metcalfe DD. Evaluation of immediate adverse reactions to foods in adult patients: Part 1: correlation of demographic, laboratory, and prick skin test data with response to controlled oral food challenge. J Allergy Clin Immunol. 1985;75:348–55.

Sachs M, Yunginer JW. Food-induced anaphylaxis. Immunol Allergy Clin North Am. 1991;11:743–55.

Sampson HA. Differential diagnosis in adverse reactions to foods. J Allergy Clin Immunol. 1986;78:212–9.

Latex Allergy

Kelly KJ, Kurup V, Zacharisen M, et al. Skin and serologic resting in the diagnosis of latex allergy. J Allergy Clin Immunol. 1993;91:1140–45.

Kurup VP, Kelly KJ, Turjanmaa K, et al. Immunoglobulin E reactivity to latex antigens in the sera of patients from Finland and the United States. J Allergy Clin Immunol. 1993;91:1128–34.

Moneret-Vautrin DA, Beaudouin E, Widmer S, et al. Prospective study of risk factors in natural rubber latex hypersensitivity. J Allergy Clin Immunol. 1993;92:668–77.

Task Force on Allergic Reactions to Latex. Committee report. J Allergy Clin Immunol. 1993;92:16–8.

Exercise-Induced Allergy

Horan RF, Sheffer AL. Exercise-induced anaphylaxis. Immunol Allergy Clin North Am. 1992;12:559-69.

Contrast Media Allergy

Greenberger P. Contrast media reactions. J Allergy Clin Immunol. 1984;74:600–5.

Lasser EC, Berry CC, Talner LB, et al. Pretreatment with corticosteroids to alleviate reactions to intravenous contrast material. N Engl J Med. 1985;317:845–9.

Shehadi WH. Contrast media adverse reactions: occurrence, recurrence, and distribution patterns. Radiology. 1982;143:11–7.

Aspirin Allergy

Stevenson DD. Aspirin and nonsteroidal anti-inflammatory drugs. Immunol Allergy Clin North Am. 1995;15:529–52.

Stevenson DD, Hankammer MA, Mathison DA, et al. Aspirin desensitization treatment of aspirin-sensitive patients with rhinosinusitis-asthma: long term outcomes. J Allergy Clin Immunol. 1996;98:751–8.

Idiopathic Allergy

Orfan NA, Stoloff RS, Harris KE, et al. Idiopathic anaphylaxis: total experience with 225 patients. Allergy Proc. 1992;12:35–43.

Patterson R, Hogan M, Yarnold P, et al. Idiopathic anaphylaxis. Arch Int Med. 1995; 155:869–71.

Chapter 7

Drug Allergy

Mark S. Dykewicz, MD

Adverse drug reactions are the most common iatrogenic illnesses, estimated to occur during 1% to 15% of drug therapy courses. Fatal drug reactions have an estimated prevalence of 0.10% for medical inpatients and 0.01% for surgical inpatients. The majority of adverse drug reactions result from nonimmunologic or unknown mechanisms, such as toxic overdose, drug interactions, or idiosyncratic intolerance (Table 7.1). Approximately 5% to 10% are caused by proven or suspected immunologic mechanisms (Box 7.1). Immunologic drug reactions are mediated by specific antibodies, sensitized T cells, or both, that develop because of sensitization induced by previous or continuous exposure to the same or antigenically related drug. The diagnosis of an immunologic drug reaction is often based on clinical presentation, although identification of antibodies or sensitized T cells directed against the drug may help confirm the diagnosis.

Factors Influencing the Development of Immunologic Drug Reactions

The risk for development of drug reactions may be influenced by factors related to drug administration and inherent characteristics of the drug and host.

Table 7.1 Categories of Nonimmunologic Adverse Drug Reactions

Category	Description	Example
Toxic overdose	Excessive dose or impaired secretion	Convulsions from overdose of lidocaine leads to toxic effects
Toxic side effects	Therapeutically undesirable pharmacologic action that may occur at normal drug doses	Drowsiness from antihistamines
Intolerance or idiosyncrasy	Quantitatively abnormal response that may be similar to or different from pharmacologic effects; may involve enzyme deficiencies	Hemolytic anemia from sulfa drugs in glucose-6-phosphate dehydrogenase deficiency
Secondary drug effect	Drug effect unrelated to primary pharmacologic action	Diuretic effect of theophylline
Drug interaction	Action of a drug on effectiveness or toxicity of another drug	Theophylline toxicity caused by reduced hepatic clearance from use of cimetidine
Drug teratogenicity	Drugs used during pregnancy causing fetal defects	Hypoplastic limb formation from thalidomide
Maternal–fetal toxic drug transfer	Toxic effects on fetus or newborn from drugs taken by mother	Narcotic effects on newborns
Superinfection	Promotion of infection secondary to antibacterial action of drugs	Clostridium difficile pseudomembranous colitis from broad-spectrum antibiotics
Jarisch–Herxheimer reaction	Release of microbial antigens or endotoxins caused by bacterial effects of antibiotics	Fever, chills, and localized edema from penicillin therapy for syphilis
Cytokine-release syndrome	Release of cytokines caused by effects of biologic agents	Fever, chills, and rigors after infusion of antilymphocyte antibodies

Modified from Condemi JJ and Dykewicz MS, eds. Allergy and Immunology Medical Knowledge Self-Assessment Program (MKSAP). 2nd ed. Philadelphia: American College of Physicians; 1997.

Dosage and Exposure

Multiple, intermittent exposures to a drug increase the risk of allergic reactions to that drug, particularly IgE-mediated reactions; however, increasing intervals between courses of a drug decrease the risk of an allergic reaction. Higher drug doses may increase the risks of some kinds of drug reactions, such as hemolytic anemia from penicillin. Allergic reactions that develop during a course of drug administration (e.g., skin rashes, serum sickness) are more frequently observed in the early weeks of a drug course and become less common with continued drug administration.

Box 7.1 Allergic, Presumed Immunologic, and Anaphylactoid Reactions to Drugs

Reactions conforming to Gell and Coombs mechanisms

Type I

   IgE-mediated, immediate-type hypersensitivity (anaphylaxis from penicillin, insulin)

Type II

   Cytotoxic antibody (hemolytic anemia, thrombocytopenia, granulocytopenia from penicillin, α-methyldopa)

Type III

   Antibody–antigen immune complex (serum sickness from penicillin or heterologous antisera)

Type IV

   Delayed-type, cell-mediated hypersensitivity (contact dermatitis from neomycin)

Allergic reactions presumed to be immunologic but not conforming to Gell and Coombs classification

Drug-associated skin eruptions

Febrile mucocutaneous syndromes

   Stevens–Johnson syndrome

   Lyell syndrome

Drug fever

Pulmonary infiltrates with eosinophilia

Eosinophilic myocarditis

Interstitial nephritis

Nephrotic syndrome

Hepatocellular, cholestatic, and granulomatous liver reaction

Generalized lymphadenopathy

Aseptic meningitis

Anaphylactoid reactions

Non–IgE-mediated, immediate-type anaphylactoid reactions

   Radiographic contrast media

   Aspirin and nonsteroidal anti-inflammatory drugs

   Narcotics

Modified from Condemi JJ, Dykewicz MS, eds. Allergy and Immunology Medical Knowledge Self-Assessment Program (MKSAP), 2nd ed. Philadelphia: American College of Physicians; 1997.

Route

The route of drug administration can alter the risk and presentation of an immunologic reaction. Parenteral (intravenous or intramuscular) administration of penicillin is more likely to cause sensitization and subsequent anaphylaxis than is oral administration. When anaphylaxis does occur from oral administration, however, it is more likely to have a prolonged course, possibly reflecting prolonged, delayed absorption. Inhalation of drugs to which one is immunologically sensitized generally causes reactions limited to upper respiratory or conjunctival manifestations, although severe asthma and anaphylaxis can occur (e.g., psyllium).

Structure of Compound

Higher molecular weight compounds (> 5000 D) and those of greater structural complexity (e.g., proteins from nonhuman sources) are more likely to induce immunologic responses and allergic reactions. The ability of many smaller molecular weight compounds (e.g., most antibiotics) to induce allergic reactions is dependent on their ability to serve as haptens as they conjugate to self proteins. Drugs such as β-lactam antibiotics, which readily react with self proteins, become covalently bound to self-protein carriers, such as human serum albumin, to form antigenic conjugates. Many non–β-lactam antibiotics cannot react directly with self-protein carriers but must be metabolized by hepatic cytochrome P_{450} or other enzyme systems to form reactive products that then bind with self-protein carriers. Consequently, performing skin testing or in vitro testing with the parent drug may not identify relevant immunologic sensitivity to a reactive intermediate product.

Although the incidence of immunologic reactions to human proteins used as drugs is usually low, reactions may occur, in part because of the body's well recognized capacity for mounting autoimmune responses against native proteins. Conformational changes of tertiary protein structure that develop during manufacturing or purification processes can confer allergenicity, even to recombinant human proteins such as insulin.

Host Factors

Host factors influence the risk of allergic drug reactions. Children have a lower risk for developing allergic drug reactions than adults, reflecting either age-related differences between the pediatric and adult immune systems or the relatively smaller cumulative exposure of children to drugs. When normalized for the number of drugs received, age, and diagnosis, women have an incidence of cutaneous drug reactions that is 35% higher than that in men. Atopic individuals had been thought to be at higher risk for serious drug reactions, but the incidence of positive skin-test reactivity to penicillin is the same for atopic and nonatopic patients. Cystic fibrosis patients have a high rate of drug reactions that cannot be fully explained by their repetitive exposure to multiple medications. Genetic factors may influence the risk of allergic drug reactions, e.g., the HLA-DR3 phenotype has been linked to insulin allergy in diabetics and to nephropathy in patients treated with penicillamine or gold for rheumatoid arthritis. Seriously ill patients and those who have received multiple courses of drugs develop allergic drug reactions more frequently, although there is no correlation between the incidence of cutaneous drug reactions and advanced age, diagnosis, or survival. During infections, immune system upregulation can occur, promoting immune responses to new antigens, including drugs. Cytokine responses during infections may vary between individuals, but there is usually production and release of interleukin (IL)-1, IL-6, tumor necrosis factor, and other cytokines that can promote immune effector systems. It has been proposed that bacterial killing from administration of antibiotics can release endotoxins that also cause release and production of cytokines. Whether an individual is a rapid or slow metabolizer of a drug may alter production of immunogenic reactive intermediates and thereby influence the likelihood of developing immunologic drug reactions.

A multiple drug allergy syndrome has been reported in patients with a history of penicillin allergic reactions (e.g., anaphylaxis, urticaria, angioedema) who have a history of reactions to drugs that are antigenically unrelated to penicillins (e.g., erythromycin). Reactions (e.g., maculopapular rashes) to the nonpenicillin drugs can differ from reactions to penicillins. Consequently, the tendency for some individuals to develop multiple drug allergies cannot be explained as simply an HLA-associated genetic propensity to produce IgE to drugs.

Although the mechanism is not completely understood, approximately 50% of AIDS patients treated with trimethoprim-sulfamethoxazole for *Pneumocystis carinii* infection develop drug rashes—a 10-fold higher incidence than that observed in those with normal immune status. AIDS patients also have an increased incidence of drug fever, neutropenia, and thrombocytopenia from sulfa drugs and higher rates of adverse reactions to rifampin, dapsone, and other antibiotics.

Classification of Drug Reactions by Mechanism and Temporal Course

Immunologic drug reactions may be classified either by the presumptive immunologic mechanism responsible for the reaction or by the temporal relation between drug exposure and the appearance of adverse manifestations. When confronted with an adverse immunologic drug reaction in a patient, classifying the reaction by these schemes may aid in making clinical decisions about evaluation and management.

Gell and Coombs Classification

The Gell and Coombs classification (*see* Box 7.1) defines four basic immunologic mechanisms responsible for reactions, although not all drug reactions suspected to have an immunologic basis conform to this system (e.g., nonurticarial drug rashes). In an individual patient, several mechanisms may be operative simultaneously.

Type I

Type I (immunoglobulin E–mediated hypersensitivity) reactions occur when IgE antibodies that are bound to the surface of mast cells or basophils recognize and bind to a drug antigen, thereby causing cross-linking of adjacent IgE antibodies, with consequent cell activation and release of mediators such as histamine, tryptase, and leukotrienes. In full expression, generalized anaphylaxis develops, although any of the manifestations of anaphylaxis (e.g., pruritus, flushing, urticaria, angioedema, laryngeal edema, bronchospasm, rhinoconjunctivitis, hypotension, tachycardia, nausea, vomiting, diarrhea, abdominal and uterine cramps) may occur singly or in combination. Usually type I reactions occur within seconds to minutes of parenteral drug administration, although they may develop up to several hours after oral administration. Common causes of type I reactions include antibiotics, proteins (e.g., antisera, insulin and other peptide hormones, chymopapain, streptokinase), vaccines, and allergen extracts.

Anaphylaxis must be distinguished from other causes of syncope or vascular collapse, most notably vasovagal reactions that may occur after any traumatic procedure, including injection. A vasovagal reaction typically presents with diaphoresis, blanching (rather than flushing), nausea, and rapid improvement with recumbency. Although hypotension may be present in both conditions, bradycardia occurs more frequently in vasovagal reactions, whereas tachycardia is more typical of anaphylaxis. Anaphylactoid reactions have clinical presentations that are similar to those of IgE-mediated anaphylaxis, but they are caused by mast cell mediator release or complement activation without involvement of IgE antibody. Anaphylactoid reactions may be caused by a variety of agents, including radiographic contrast media, aspirin and nonsteroidal anti-inflammatory drugs (NSAIDs), and narcotics.

Type II

Type II (cytotoxic/cytolytic) reactions occur when IgG or IgM antibodies recognize a drug antigen associated with cell membranes or a cross-reactive cell-membrane antigen (e.g., a blood group antigen or platelet membrane glycoprotein); consequent interaction with the complement causes cell destruction. Examples of these reactions include immune hemolytic anemia and thrombocytopenia from penicillins and quinidine.

Type III

Type III (immune-complex) reactions occur when a drug combines with antibodies (usually IgG or IgM) to form immune complexes that are deposited within blood vessel walls and basement membranes, leading to tissue damage. Circulating immune complexes cause serum sickness reactions that may include fever, skin lesions (e.g., urticaria, angioedema, maculopapular or morbilliform rashes, palpable purpura), lymphadenopathy, arthralgias, nephritis, and hepatitis. Generally, serum sickness occurs 1 to 4 weeks after drug use, but it may develop several days after administration if there has been previous exposure to the agent. Type III immune-complex mechanisms may also cause drug-induced lupus syndromes from hydralazine, procainamide, isoniazid, phenytoin, and other drugs. Unlike idiopathic systemic lupus erythematosus, it is rare for patients with drug-induced lupus to be black or to have renal involvement or anti–double-stranded DNA. Most patients with drug-induced lupus have antibodies to histone. In the case of drug-induced lupus syndromes, clinical symptoms usually abate within weeks after cessation of the causative drug, but a positive antihistone antinuclear antibodies test may persist for months to years.

Subcutaneous or intramuscular injection of drug antigens (e.g., insulin, nonhuman antisera) may cause local induration of the skin that is characterized by a neutrophilic infiltrate and termed an *Arthus reaction*. The reaction develops because of in situ formation of immune complexes that develop when preexisting antibody binds with injected drug antigen.

Type IV

Type IV (delayed hypersensitivity) reactions are mediated by sensitized lymphocytes. Allergic contact dermatitis is a classic example of a type IV reaction. This frequently develops 24 to 72 hours after topical application of a drug, although during first presentation, the interval between exposure and development of dermatitis may be 1 week. Local anesthetic agents, paraben preservatives, topical aminoglycosides, and ethylenediamine (used as a stabilizer in dermatologic preparations) are examples of agents that cause contact dermatitis. Subcutaneous injection of drugs may cause induration through a type IV mechanism.

Classification of Drug Reactions by Temporal Course

Whatever the immunologic mechanism, all drug reactions can be categorized as being one of three types (i.e., immediate, accelerated, and delayed or late reactions), depending on the temporal onset of manifestations in relation to drug administration.

Immediate reactions occur within the first hour after drug administration and include manifestations of anaphylaxis. Accelerated reactions occur from 1 to 72 hours after administration and may manifest as exanthems, fever, urticaria, nonurticarial rashes, or angioedema. Delayed or late reactions occur 72 hours or more after administration and may manifest as urticarial and nonurticarial rashes, serum sickness–like reactions, fever, or a variety of cardiopulmonary, hematologic, hepatic, renal, and vasculitic reactions.

Clinical Patterns of Drug Eruptions

Although some drugs cause atypical reactions not generally elicited by other agents, most drugs cause adverse drug reactions that have well-described clinical patterns that may be caused by myriad drugs. Adverse drug reactions may involve nearly all organs of the body. Although immunologic drug reactions frequently improve within several days after stopping the causative drug, some drug reactions may increase in severity weeks after drug cessation (e.g., serum sickness–like reactions).

Skin Eruptions

The most common manifestations of drug reactions involve the skin. These may present as maculopapular, morbilliform or erythematous rashes, urticaria and angioedema, erythema multiforme, erythema nodosum, bullous eruptions, and exfoliation. Typically, skin reactions occur several days or weeks into a drug course (although they may develop even several weeks after cessation of the responsible drug) and have symmetric distribution that initially involves the trunk but may extend to involve the extremities. Palm and sole involvement is more typical of infectious exanthems and is a helpful distinguishing characteristic. Fever and pruritus are common, but contrary to common belief, eosinophilia is frequently absent. The mechanisms of nonurticarial drug rashes are incompletely understood but do not appear to be explained by antibody-mediated mechanisms or by a classic type IV reaction. Mechanisms involving nonhumoral, cell-mediated immunity have been suggested by the association of several immunologic abnormalities, including lymphocytic skin infiltrates and increased numbers of Langerhans' cells in lesional skin. In vitro studies reveal drug-induced proliferation of peripheral blood lymphocytes (correlating best with rashes from antiseizure medications but correlating variably or poorly with sulfonamide rashes), T-cell cytokine production in response to causative drugs, and the culturing of drug-reactive lymphocyte clones from peripheral blood (found in only a minority of patients reactive to sulfonamides).

Fixed drug eruptions, which are caused by phenolphthalein and other drugs, develop in discrete regions of the skin. On repeat administration of the responsible drug, a skin eruption will recur at the same location.

After the administration of a variety of drugs, ultraviolet light exposure may induce two forms of photosensitive skin reactions. Phototoxic reactions (e.g., to tetracycline) are nonimmunologic reactions that may occur upon first exposure to a drug. They typically present as a severe sunburn and develop 4 to 8 hours after light exposure. Photoallergic reactions (e.g., to sulfonamides) are immunologically mediated reactions that are caused by ultraviolet alteration of the drug, which promotes conjugation of reactive drug intermediates to self proteins and consequent T-cell–mediated immune responses. Photoallergic rashes typically appear as an eczematous rash and occur only after days or months of drug exposure. Neither type of photosensitive reaction is associated with a significantly higher risk for other types of adverse reactions to the causative drug.

Drug Fever

Fever may present as the only manifestation of a drug reaction or may occur in concert with other manifestations of drug reactions. The usual mechanism for a febrile response to a drug is the release of pyrogens from phagocytes, following either phagocytic engulfment of drug–IgG immune complexes or phagocytic stimulation by cytokines released from sensitized T cells. Drug fever generally occurs 7 to 10 days into a drug course, although it may occur earlier or later. Clinically, a disparity between the degree of fever and patient well-being may help to identify fever as drug induced. There should be prompt defervescence (within 48 h) when the causative drug is stopped.

Internal Organ Involvement

Adverse drug reactions may involve internal organs, resulting in systemic vasculitic syndromes; interstitial nephritis; nephrotic syndrome; hepatocellular, cholestatic, or granulomatous hepatic reactions; eosinophilic myocarditis; lung disorders; and other syndromes. Generalized lymphadenopathy as the only manifestation of an adverse drug reaction has been observed with long-term treatment with penicillin, phenytoin, and sulfonamides.

Many drugs (e.g., penicillins, carbamazepine, and the sulfonamides) have been reported to cause the pulmonary infiltrates with eosinophilia syndrome. Generally, there is an acute onset of a nonproductive cough within 10 days of the start of drug administration. This is associated with chest discomfort, malaise, headache, migratory infiltrates on chest radiograph, and peripheral eosinophilia.

Most cases of pulmonary fibrosis caused by drugs are due to toxic, nonimmune mechanisms (e.g., bleomycin, methysergide), but immunologic mechanisms are probably important in other cases.

Aseptic meningitis has been reported from NSAIDs, antithymocyte globulin, and intravenous immunoglobulin (IVIG). Cases of aseptic meningitis from IVIG are typical in that illnesses usually begin 12 to 24 hours after administration, and recovery generally ensues within several days after withdrawal of the medication. Patients present with severe headache, meningeal signs, and photophobia. Most cases have abnormal cerebrospinal fluid findings, including leukocytosis (predominantly neutrophilic) and elevated protein.

Febrile Mucocutaneous Syndromes

Drug reactions, infections (e.g., Herpes simplex, *Mycoplasma pneumoniae*), or idiopathic causes may result in a spectrum of febrile mucocutaneous syndromes that involve the skin and mucous membranes, cause exfoliation, and damage internal organs (including the gastrointestinal and respiratory tracts), with a consequent significant risk of infection and fatality. These syndromes include Stevens–Johnson syndrome (erythema multiforme or other skin eruptions with mucous membrane involvement) and toxic epidermal necrolysis or Lyell syndrome (bullous skin disease that may include mucositis). Stevens–Johnson syndrome may cause permanent ocular damage. Skin biopsy differentiates subepidermal cleavage that is characteristic of drug-induced toxic epidermal necrolysis from intraepidermal cleavage that is characteristic of the scalded-skin syndrome induced by staphylococcal toxins. Drugs associated with the febrile mucocutaneous syndromes include sulfonamides, penicillins, phenytoin, and phenobarbital. The mechanism of these syndromes is uncertain. Although corticosteroid administration late in the course of febrile mucocutaneous syndromes has been reported to be associated with higher morbidity, some authorities advocate early use of corticosteroids to prevent progression and fatality. Readministration of or attempted desensitization to a drug incriminated in causing Stevens–Johnson syndrome should not be attempted because of the risk of recurrent Stevens–Johnson syndrome and fatality.

Specific Drugs Causing Hypersensitivity Reactions

General Anesthetic Agents

During anesthesia, anaphylactoid reactions may be caused by muscle relaxants (e.g., succinylcholine, alcuronium, pancuronium, fluphenazine, gallamine, D-tubocurarine), induction agents (e.g., thiopental, propanidid), opiates, or antibiotics. Although histamine release has been implicated in the pathogenesis of some reactions from induction agents and muscle relaxants, the responsible mechanism for many reactions is not established. Quaternary ammonium muscle relaxants (e.g., succinylcholine) can cause systemic reactions through IgE and non–IgE-mediated mechanisms. Consequently, negative skin tests to these agents cannot reliably predict safe administration. Narcotics generally cause release of mediators, such as histamine, by non–IgE-mediated mechanisms via direct effects on mast cells, although rare IgE-mediated reactions have been reported.

Local Anesthetic Agents

The majority of adverse reactions from local anesthetic agents are toxic reactions caused by rapid drug absorption, inadvertent intravenous injection, or overdosage. Toxic reactions typically target the cardiovascular and central nervous systems and may include hypotension, cardiorespiratory failure, and convulsions. Epinephrine—commonly present in local anesthetic preparations to prolong duration of anesthesia—is often responsible for adverse effects, such as shakiness or tachycardia. Urticaria, angioedema, and anaphylactoid idiosyncratic reactions rarely occur from local anesthetics and, except for one or two case reports, are likely not IgE mediated. Delayed-type lymphocytic reactivity is responsible for contact dermatitis and for some large local reactions from local anesthetics. There is immunologic cross-reactivity for delayed-type hypersensitivity among so-called group I agents (esters of benzoic acid, e.g., procaine/Novocaine, tetracaine/Pontocaine) but not among group II agents (non-ester/amides of benzoic acid, e.g., lidocaine/Xylocaine, mepivacaine/Carbocaine, bupivacaine/Marcaine) nor between group I and group II agents. Parabens, which are used as preservatives in cosmetics and in topical therapeutic agents, have chemical structures similar to group I agents, but there are conflicting data about whether there is significant immunologic cross-reactivity.

In cases of suspected local anesthetic allergy, the usual approach is to test the dose with a subcutaneous injection of the local anesthetic agent to be used (Table 7.2). The choice of the agent to be tested and administered is based upon 1) the history of the previous reaction (with readministration being relatively contraindicated if the reaction was serious and unlikely to have occurred through inadvertent intravenous administration), 2) the local anesthetic agent preferred by the dentist or surgeon, and 3) the preference for use of a group II agent when a group I agent was suspected of having caused the previous reaction. Some authorities prefer to precede subcutaneous test dosing with prick or intradermal skin tests; others avoid intradermal skin tests because they may induce false-positive irritant responses. Because the vaso-

Table 7.2 Local Anesthetic Provocative Dose Testing

Route	Dilution	Dose
Prick test*	Undiluted	I drop
Intradermal test*	1:100	0.02 mL
Subcutaneous challenge†	1:100	0.10 mL
Subcutaneous	1:10	0.10 mL
Subcutaneous	Undiluted	0.10 mL
Subcutaneous	Undiluted	1.00 mL
Subcutaneous (optional)	Undiluted	2.00 mL

* Skin test with local anesthetic (free of epinephrine/parabens); as discussed in text, some would forego intradermal testing.
† Challenge with the local anesthetic (negative on skin test) sequentially at 15-min intervals as recommended by de Shazo and Nelson.
Modified from Anderson JA. Allergic reactions to drugs and biologic agents. JAMA. 1992;286:2845–58.

constrictive action of epinephrine may reduce local reactions from local anesthetic agents and therefore confound interpretation of subcutaneous test dosing, the local anesthetic preparation used for test dosing must not contain epinephrine.

Case 7.1

A 73-year-old man had four episodes of angioedema over the last 2 months. Angioedema had involved the face, tongue, lips, and hands. The episodes were without clear relation to food ingestion, exercise, or trauma. He was treated with hydroxyzine and prednisone for each episode, with slow resolution of swelling over several days. These episodes were not been associated with urticaria, respiratory complaints, light-headedness, nausea, or vomiting.

The patient had a history of hypertension and smokes tobacco. Eight months ago, he had an anterior myocardial infarction (MI) complicated by mild congestive heart failure; however, while on his current medication regimen, he has had minimal symptoms of angina and no evidence of congestive heart failure.

The patient was taking metoprolol for several years for his hypertension. During hospitalization for his MI, he was begun on lisinopril, furosemide, and aspirin 81 mg/d.

The most likely cause of angioedema in this patient is the use of an angiotensin-converting–enzyme (ACE) inhibitor (lisinopril). ACE-inhibitor–induced angioedema may not begin until after many months of medication use, and then occurs only episodically, even though the medication is taken on a daily basis. In contrast, angioedema and urticaria from aspirin or other drugs will typically occur on a daily basis once sensitivity develops. Most patients who develop ACE-inhibitor–induced angioedema (or even more commonly cough) can tolerate angiotensin-II–receptor antagonists, which provide many of the beneficial hemodynamic effects of ACE inhibitors.

Angiotensin-Converting–Enzyme Inhibitors

Well-described adverse effects of ACE inhibitors include cough (incidence in up to 25% of patients), increased nasal mucus production and postnasal drip, and angioedema (incidence, 0.1%–0.2%). Generally, cough and angioedema do not occur in the same patient. ACE-inhibitor–induced cough has an onset from 1 day to 12 months after initiation of therapy and may be associated with increased bronchial hyperreactivity to methacholine. After discontinuation of ACE inhibitors, cough disappears within 1 to 2 weeks in most patients, although it may persist for several more weeks. Angioedema commonly involves the face and oral pharyngeal tissues; involvement of the latter may result in life-threatening airway obstruction. Although ACE-inhibitor angioedema frequently develops within the first week of therapy, it can develop even after many months of administration. Patients with a history of idiopathic angioedema have been reported to develop more severe and frequent episodes of angioedema when taking ACE inhibitors. There have been rare reports that ACE inhibitors have caused abdominal pain and ascites from angioedema of the abdominal viscera. Intolerance to one ACE inhibitor is generally associated with intolerance to all drugs of this class. There is no evidence that a classic immunologic mechanism is responsible for these reactions; hence, skin testing has no value. By inhibiting ACE (also known as kininase II), ACE inhibitors promote the accumulation of bradykinin and other vasoactive peptides, which in part may account for the side effects due to ACE inhibitors. Most of the beneficial pharmacologic effects of ACE inhibitors are thought to result from reduction of the ACE-catalyzed conversion of angiotensin I to angiotensin II (a vasoconstrictor and stimulator of aldosterone secretion). Angiotensin-II–receptor antagonists (e.g., losarten, valsarten) appear to possess desirable cardiovascular effects similar to ACE inhibitors but can be tolerated by most patients who develop cough or angioedema from ACE inhibitors.

β-Lactam Antibiotics

Penicillins

Penicillin antibiotics are among the most common causes of immunologic drug reactions, including those mediated by all four Gell and Coombs mechanisms, delayed maculopapular rashes, drug fever, mucocutaneous syndromes (e.g., Stevens–Johnson syndrome), acute interstitial nephritis, and pulmonary infiltrates with eosinophilia. The incidence of immunologic reactions to penicillin does not appear to be affected by sex, race, or HLA phenotype. A non-immunologic rash is frequently seen with ampicillin and amoxicillin and has an increased incidence with concomitant viral infections (e.g., Epstein–Barr syndrome), chronic lymphocytic leukemia, hyperuricemia, and allopurinol administration. These rashes, which are generally nonpruritic in contrast to immunologically mediated rashes, are not associated with an increased risk for future immunologic reactions to penicillin antibiotics. Immediate-type reactions, including anaphylaxis, are less common with antistaphylococcal penicillins (e.g., dicloxacillin, methicillin, nafcillin) and antipseudomonal penicillins (e.g., carbenicillin, piperacillin, ticarcillin). Acute interstitial nephritis is more frequently associated with methicillin. Amoxicillin, in combination with the β-lactamase inhibitor clavulanic acid, has been associated with cholestatic jaundice, but clavulanic acid may be responsible for many of these reactions.

IgE-antibody–mediated systemic reactions occur during approximately 2% of penicillin courses, and of those reactions, up to 10% are life threatening. Anaphylactic reactions to penicillins most commonly occur in adults between 20 and 49 years of age. Most fatalities from anaphylaxis to penicillins occur in patients with no history of penicillin allergy. Patients with previous systemic IgE-mediated reactions to penicillin are at increased risk for both IgE-mediated and non-IgE–mediated reactions on subsequent administrations. Patients with an IgE-mediated reaction to penicillins tend to lose their sensitivity if there is no further drug exposure. After an immediate reaction to penicillin, 50% of patients are skin-test negative 5 years later, and 75% to 80% are skin-test negative after 10 years. There is evidence, however, that patients who have lost penicillin sensitivity may be more likely to be sensitized by subsequent administration of penicillin than the general population.

Most immunologic reactions to penicillins are directed against β-lactam core determinants. Approximately 95% of penicillin is metabolized to form the benzylpenicilloyl (BPO) moiety—referred to as the *major determinant*. Although the BPO major determinant is only occasionally responsible for severe, IgE-mediated, immediate reactions, IgE antibodies to the major determinant are usually responsible for accelerated reactions (1–72 h after penicillin administration) and delayed or late urticaria (> 72 h after administration). Circulating immune complexes of IgG to BPO have been associated with serum-sickness reactions, and IgM and IgG antibodies to BPO have been associated with Coombs-positive hemolytic anemia from penicillin. Although less than 5% of penicillin is metabolized to the *minor determinants* (which include benzyl penicillin G, penicilloates, and benzylpenicilloylamine), IgE antibodies to the minor determinants are usually responsible for severe immediate-type reactions to penicillin.

Skin testing with both penicillin G and a stabilized major determinant preparation (benzylpenicilloyl-polylysine, Pre-Pen, Schwarz Pharma) identifies approximately 90% to 93% of patients at risk for immediate reactions to penicillins. The addition of testing with a minor determinant mixture significantly increases the negative predictive value of penicillin skin testing. Only 0.5% to 3.0% of patients who are skin-test negative to major and minor determinants have adverse reactions compatible with IgE-mediated immediate or accelerated penicillin allergy, and none of these reactions has been reported to be fatal or life threatening. Unfortunately, a penicillin minor-determinant mixture is not yet commercially available. Although skin testing with these penicillin core determinants can generally detect patients at risk for immediate reactions to semisynthetic penicillins, this is not absolute because IgE antibodies to side-chain determinants unique to semisynthetic penicillins may cause reactions. Although reactivity to side-chain determinants of semisynthetic penicillins is considered uncommon in the general population, this may not be true in special high-risk groups. One report indicates that 20% of cystic fibrosis patients who are at risk for IgE-mediated reactions to semisynthetic penicillins can be detected only by skin testing with semisynthetic penicillin determinants. Nonetheless, skin testing to side-chain determinants is not commonly performed in the general population, and the predictive value of such testing has not been fully established.

Who Should Undergo Penicillin Skin Testing? Patients with a history of anaphylaxis, urticaria, or serum sickness associated with penicillin use should be skin tested before administration of penicillin.

Patients with a history of bullous skin eruptions and exfoliative dermatitis (including Stevens–Johnson syndrome and toxic epidermal necrolysis) from penicillin should not be skin tested and should not receive penicillin antibiotics because of the risk of potentially life-threatening recurrent reactions.

Patients with a history of maculopapular or morbilliform skin rashes to penicillin may be considered for skin testing, but some evidence suggests that such patients generally are not at high risk for developing immediate-type reactions.

Patients with a positive family history but no personal history of penicillin allergy generally do not need to undergo skin testing, because a positive family history does not predict a reaction rate greater than the general population.

In vitro radioallergosorbent tests and enzyme-linked immunosorbent assays can detect IgE antibody to the major determinant, but these tests are unable to identify all patients who have positive skin tests to the major determinant. Moreover, in vitro tests to minor determinants are not available in clinical practice. Consequently, the clinical usefulness of in vitro testing to identify penicillin allergy is limited, although a patient should be considered at increased risk for a reaction if an in vitro test for IgE antibody to the major determinant is positive.

Depending on the patient's clinical history of allergy and available skin or in vitro test results for IgE to penicillin determinants and the necessity to use a penicillin antibiotic, various protocols of test dosing or desensitization to penicillin may be employed. If penicillin skin testing is positive (identifying the patient as being at increased risk for anaphylaxis) and there is an essential or compelling indication to use a penicillin antibiotic, rapid desensitization protocols should be used (Tables 7.3 and 7.4). If the skin test is negative (indicating that the patient is not at significant current risk for an immediate-type reaction) and the patient had a prior history of an immediate-type reaction (e.g., anaphylaxis, urticaria), the patient may receive penicillin without desensitization, although some physicians might precede full-dose administration with a small test dose if the previous reaction was life threatening.

Cephalosporins

Cephalosporins, like penicillins, cause a wide variety of adverse immunologic reactions. Third-generation cephalosporins (e.g., cefotaxime, moxalactam) have a lower incidence of immediate-type reactions than do first-generation (e.g., cefaclor, cephalexin, cephaloridine, cephalothin, cephradine) or second-generation (e.g., cefoxitin, cefamandole) cephalosporins. Nonimmunologic disulfiram-like reactions (e.g., flushing, hypotension, nausea, vomiting, respiratory distress) may occur in patients drinking alcohol after administration of cephalosporins containing a 3-methylthiotetrazole side chain (e.g., cefoperazone). Allergic reactions to cephalosporins may occur in the absence of penicillin allergy, apparently due to antigenic determinants unique to cephalosporins. There is evidence that for some cephalosporins, side chains (e.g., the 2-thiophene group and the attached-methylene group of cephalothin) are important allergenic determinants. In general, side-chain determinants are more important in cephalosporin allergy than in penicillin allergy. Currently, skin testing for cephalosporin allergy is experimental.

Both penicillins and cephalosporins contain a β-lactam ring as part of a bicyclic nucleus (which accounts for undisputed in vitro allergenic cross-reactivity between them) and an amide side chain (Fig. 7.1). There are, however, conflicting data about the degree of clinically significant cross-reactivity between these drug classes, and a few authorities assert that there is no significant clinical cross-reactivity. Skin-testing studies have reported 30% to 70% cross reactivity between positive skin tests to penicillin determinants and first-generation cephalosporins, such as cephalothin. In one large study of patients who had a history of penicillin reactions, the risk of allergic reactions to various cephalosporins was 8.1%, which is an approximately fourfold greater reaction rate than for patients with a history of no reaction to penicillin. However, because penicillin-allergic patients appear to be at increased risk for allergic reactions to even structurally unrelated drugs, the contribution of β-lactam cross-reactivity to the increased risk for reactions to first-generation cephalosporins in penicillin-allergic patients cannot be assessed. Available evidence indicates that penicillin allergic patients are at less risk for allergic reactions to second- and third-generation cephalosporins than to first-generation cephalosporins. Many allergist–immunologists currently recommend caution or avoidance of cephalosporins in patients with known sensitivity to penicillins, particularly if there is a history of immediate-type sensitivity reactions.

Table 7.3 β-Lactam Oral Desensitization Protocol

Dose No.*	Stock Concentration (mg/mL) †	Volume (mL)	Dose (mg)	Cumulative Drug (mg)
1	0.5	0.05	0.025	0.025
2	0.5	0.10	0.050	0.075
3	0.5	0.20	0.100	0.175
4	0.5	0.40	0.200	0.375
5	0.5	0.80	0.400	0.775
6	5.0	0.15	0.750	1.525
7	5.0	0.30	1.500	3.025
8	5.0	0.60	3.000	6.025
9	5.0	1.20	6.000	12.025
10	5.0	2.40	12.000	24.025
11	50.0	0.50	25.000	49.025
12	50.0	1.20	60.000	109.025
13	50.0	2.50	125.000	234.025
14	50.0	5.00	250.000	484.025

* Oral dose is approximately doubled every 15–30 min.
† Dilutions made from 250 mg/5 mL of pediatric syrup.
Modified from Sullivan T, Yecies L, Shatz G, Parker CW, Wedner HJ. Desensitization of patients allergic to penicillin using orally administer β-lactam antibodies. J Allergy Clin Immunol. 1982; 69:275–8; and Anderson JA. Allergic reactions to drugs and biologic agents. JAMA. 1992;286:2845–58.

Carbapenems

Carbapenem antibiotics (e.g., imipenem) contain a bicyclic nucleus with a β-lactam ring (*see* Fig. 7-1) and may cause allergic reactions similar to those observed with penicillins and cephalosporins. Significant allergenic cross-reactivity (determined by in vitro tests and immediate type skin testing) has been reported between imipenem and penicillin. Skin testing with imipenem determinants is investigational.

Carbacephems

Methylene substitution for sulfur at position 1 of the cephalosporin nucleus creates carbacephems (*see* Fig. 7.1). Based upon the limited data on loracarbef—the first carbacephem antibiotic available in the United States—there may be significant cross-reactivity with cephalosporins. Preliminary data suggest cross-reactivity with cephalosporins. Carbacephem skin testing is investigational.

Monobactams

The monobactams (e.g., aztreonam) have a monocyclic β-lactam nucleus that is distinct from the bicyclic nuclei of other β-lactam classes (*see* Fig 7.1). Immune reactivity toward aztreonam is predominantly directed against side-

Table 7.4 β-Lactam Intravenous Desensitization Protocol*

Dose No.	β-Lactam Concentration (mg/mL)	Penicillin G Concentration (U/mL)	Volume Given (mL)	Dose Given (mg; U)
1	0.1	160	0.10	0.01; 16
2	0.1	160	0.20	0.02; 32
3	0.1	160	0.40	0.04; 64
4	0.1	160	0.80	0.08; 128
5	1.0	1600	0.15	0.15; 240
6	1.0	1600	0.30	0.30; 480
7	1.0	1600	0.60	0.60; 960
8	1.0	1600	1.00	1.00; 1600
9	10.0	16,000	0.20	2.00; 3200
10	10.0	16,000	0.40	4.00; 6400
11	10.0	16,000	0.80	8.00; 12,800
12	100.0	160,000	0.15	15.00; 24,000
13	100.0	160,000	0.30	30.00; 48,000
14	100.0	160,000	0.60	60.00; 96,000
15	100.0	160,000	1.00	100.00; 160,000
16	1000.0	1,600,000	0.20	200.00; 320,000
17	1000.0	1,600,000	0.40	400.00; 640,000

* Observe patient for ~15–40 min after each interval dose and 30 min after final dose.
Modified from Sullivan TJ. Drug allergy. In: Middleton E, Reed CE, Ellis EF, Adkinson NF, Yunginger JW, eds.
Allergy: Principles and Practice, 4th ed. St. Louis: Mosby; 1993:1726–46.

chain rather than nuclear determinants. The only β-lactam that has been demonstrated to have significant in vitro antibody cross-reactivity with aztreonam is ceftazidime; both share an identical side-chain. Significant clinical cross reactivity between aztreonam and other β-lactam antibiotics has not been established. Monobactam skin testing is investigational.

Sulfonamides

Sulfa drugs have a high incidence of allergic reactions (2%–10% of patients without AIDS), the most common being drug exanthems and, less commonly, urticaria and other immediate-type reactions. Sulfonamides have a high degree of allergic cross-reactivity. The drug class is metabolized principally by two pathways, hepatic N-acetylation and cytochrome P_{450} N-oxidation. Genetically slow acetylators preferentially metabolize sulfa through N-oxidation to generate reactive hydroxylamine metabolites, which conjugate with proteins to form complete antigens. Consequently, slow acetylators are at increased risk for developing allergic reactions from sulfa agents. Although the N-4-sulfanamidoyl hydroxylamine metabolite is the major sulfonamide antigenic determinant recognized by

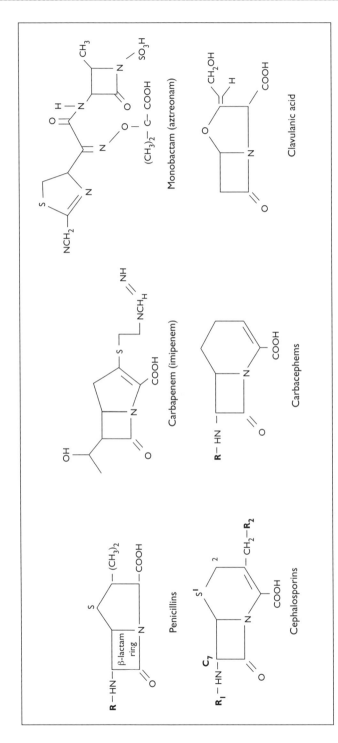

Figure 7.1 Structure of β-lactam antibiotics. Substitutions at the R position of 6-amino penicillic acid create penicillin derivatives. Substitutions at positions 1, R_1, R_2, and C_7 of 7-amino cephalosporanic acid create cephalosporin derivatives.

human IgE, a significant proportion of sulfa-sensitive patients cannot be identified by investigational skin testing using this determinant alone. Sulfasalazine, which is used for treatment of inflammatory bowel disease, contains two moieties—5-aminosalicylic acid and sulfapyridine (a sulfonamide). Most hypersensitivity reactions to this agent (e.g., rash, fever) appear to result from the sulfapyridine moiety. Slow desensitization over approximately 1 month permits tolerance of the drug in many patients who have had apparent allergic reactions. Oral and enema forms of 5-aminosalicylic acid, which is thought to be the pharmacologically active agents in sulfasalazine, are now available. These can be tolerated by 90% of patients intolerant to sulfasalazine and are effective alternative agents. A variety of slow and rapid desensitization protocols for sulfonamides have been published (Table 7.5). AIDS patients, who have a high incidence of sulfa rashes (up to 50%), can be desensitized to sulfa drugs in many cases.

Vancomycin

In addition to immunologic reactions typical of other antibiotics, vancomycin frequently is associated with nonimmunologic-infusion–related events, including hypotension, flushing, erythema, pruritus, urticaria, and pain or muscle spasms of the chest and back (red-man or red-neck syndrome). The severity of such reactions correlates with the degree of elevation of plasma histamine levels. Rapid infusion rates (> 10 mg/mL) are associated with a greater risk of severe reactions. Prospective studies have reported that 50% to 90% of patients will have some manifestations of the syndrome, although most of these are mild and of little clinical consequence. Tachyphylaxis rapidly develops in many patients, and reducing infusion rates or drug dose permits tolerance of vancomycin in most patients. One controlled study found that the H_1 antihistamine hydroxyzine (but not the H_2 antihistamine ranitidine) is beneficial in reducing erythema and pruritus from vancomycin infusions. Although uncommon compared with the frequently occurring red-man syndrome, IgE-mediated sensitivity to vancomycin can be identified by skin testing (as long as medications that interfere with skin testing, such as antihistamines or phenothiazines, have not been used).

Antibodies and Antisera

Serum sickness, anaphylactic reactions, or both may be induced by heterologous antisera, including antitoxins (e.g., for snakebite venom or botulism for which there are no human immune globulin alternatives) and antilymphocyte globulin (used for transplant rejection). The incidence of serum-sickness reactions is related to dose and occurs in almost all patients who are given a dose of antiserum greater than 100 mL. In one series, urticarial or morbilliform cu-

Table 7.5 Extended Oral Sulfasalazine Desensitization Protocol

Day	Concentration of Sulfasalazine Suspension (mg/mL)	Suspension (mL)	Sulfasalazine Dosage (mg/d)
1	1	1	1
2	1	2	2
3	1	3	4
4	1	4	8
5–11	1	10	10
12	20	1	20
13	20	2	40
14	20	4	80
15–21	20	5	100
22	20	10	200
23	20	20	400
24	20	40	800
25–31	500	2	1000 (2 tablets)
32	500	4	2000 (4 tablets)

Modified from Purdy BH, Philips DM, Summers RW. Desensitization for sulfasalazine skin rash. Ann Int Med. 1984;100:512–4.

taneous eruptions occurred in 93% of patients who developed serum sickness after administration of antithymocyte globulin. In this study, high-dose steroids did not prevent serum sickness. Many patients developed a distinctive serpiginous line of erythema, petechiae, or purpura at the margin of palmar or plantar skin. Patients who have developed serum sickness to heterologous antisera are at increased risk for developing immediate-type reactions on future readministration of antisera from the same species.

Before administering heterologous antisera to any patient, regardless of history, skin testing with antisera must be performed to detect patients at risk for anaphylaxis. Immediate-type skin testing is useful for identifying patients at risk for IgE-mediated immediate-type reactions, and desensitization to prevent immediate-type reactions may be performed when required. After desensitization to heterologous antisera, it is likely that serum sickness will develop within 8 to 12 days, but this can generally be managed successfully without long-term complications by administering both corticosteroids and regular-dosed (not as-needed) antihistamines. Immediate-type skin testing does not reliably identify patients who may develop serum sickness after administration of heterologous antisera, although patients with positive skin tests are at increased risk for developing serum sickness.

Intravenous administration of human immune serum globulin may cause immediate-type reactions by several mechanisms. Aggregation of globulins into 11S complexes may activate complement and cause anaphylaxis. An antibody to aggregated gammaglobulin has been identified in children with agam-maglobulinemia and may mediate anaphylaxis. Infusions of human immune globulin containing IgA have caused anaphylaxis in IgA-deficient patients who have developed IgE antibodies to IgA. A cytokine-release syndrome may develop in patients given infusions of heterologous or monoclonal antilym-phocyte antibodies (e.g., OKT3) for transplant rejection or lymphoid malig-nancies. The syndrome consists of fever, chills, and severe rigors during or shortly after the intravenous antibody infusion, which induces release of IL-2, interferon, and tumor necrosis factor that may be responsible for these ad-verse clinical manifestations. Infusions of antilymphocyte antibodies also cause non–IgE-mediated immediate-type reactions (e.g., urticaria, angio-edema, bronchospasm), which often occur upon first use, have a higher inci-dence in patients with lymphoid malignancies, are associated with histamine release, and cannot be predicted by skin testing.

Case 7.2

A 29-year-old woman had a history of asthma that recently was well controlled un-til last night. She had felt well yesterday and played in an evening softball game with-out respiratory complaints, but she pulled a thigh muscle while sliding into home base. Within several hours, she developed symptoms of shortness of breath and wheezing. Despite using her albuterol inhaler, she continued to have respiratory symptoms and went to the emergency room.

On physical examination, she was noted to be in some respiratory distress, with a respiratory rate of 28 and scattered wheezing. Minimal nasal polyps were noted. She was treated with β-agonists by nebulization and corticosteroids with good im-provement. After 4 hours of treatment and observation, she was discharged home.

Her asthma medications were a beclomethasone lung inhaler twice per day, a sal-meterol inhaler twice per day, and an albuterol inhaler as needed. She also took a nasal corticosteroid for a history of nasal polyps. She occasionally took aceta-minophen as needed for musculoskeletal complaints, although after her softball in-jury, she took two tablets of Alka-Seltzer Plus Sinus Medicine (which contains aspirin, brompheniramine, and phenylpropanolamine).

Approximately 1 year ago, the patient had an emergency room visit for asthma af-ter she developed "sinus" complaints for which she had taken ibuprofen. She was told to avoid taking ibuprofen, because it was suspected of contributing to her asthma exacerbation.

The most likely cause of acute asthma in this patient was the ingestion of aspirin in the over-the-counter remedy that she used for muscular complaints after the soft-ball game. This is consistent with the history of a significant asthma exacerbation in the past that was associated with ibuprofen, an NSAID that is structurally distinct

Case 7.2 (continued)

from aspirin. All NSAIDs that have significant effects on cyclo-oxygenase metabolism have the potential for causing respiratory reactions in patients who develop respiratory reactions from aspirin. Many patients who have asthma and aspirin sensitivity also have nasal polyps—the "aspirin triad" that was present in this patient.

Aspirin

Aspirin and NSAIDs may cause a variety of adverse reactions, including idiosyncratic reactions of bronchospasm, rhinitis, urticaria, angioedema, and anaphylaxis. Based upon oral challenges, aspirin sensitivity has a prevalence of 8% to 19% in adult patients with asthma and of 30% to 40% in patients with nasal polyps and sinusitis. An "aspirin triad" consisting of asthma, nasal polyps, and aspirin sensitivity may occur in some patients. Individuals with aspirin sensitivity may lose it over time.

The majority of aspirin-sensitive patients who manifest respiratory reactions, as well as some who develop urticarial reactions, have cross-sensitivity with structurally distinct NSAIDs that significantly alter arachidonic acid metabolism; however, these patients can tolerate to varying degrees NSAIDs and related compounds that have less effect on arachidonic acid metabolism (e.g., salsalate, acetaminophen at doses less than 1000 mg, and sodium and magnesium salicylate). This is consistent with the assessment that IgE-mediated sensitivity is not responsible for most cases of aspirin respiratory sensitivity or for many cases of urticarial reactions (although IgE-mediated sensitivity specific for aspirin or a particular NSAID is suspected in some cases of urticaria and anaphylaxis). Skin testing, however, is not useful. Although there are reports that some aspirin-sensitive patients develop airway obstruction following parenteral administration of corticosteroids, a link between these conditions is not certain, because similar reactions have been reported from corticosteroids in non–aspirin-sensitive asthmatics. Earlier reports that aspirin-sensitive patients have sensitivity to tartrazine (yellow dye no. 5) have not been confirmed by some double-blind challenge studies.

The mechanisms of aspirin sensitivity are not completely understood, but most evidence implicates abnormal metabolism of the arachidonic acid pathway, with increased leukotriene production. It has been theorized that cyclooxygenase blockade in aspirin-sensitive patients shunts arachidonic acid metabolites to the lipoxygenase pathway, with consequent increased production of leukotrienes and decreased production of cyclooxygenase products, such as prostaglandins and thromboxanes. Although there is evidence for enhanced generation of leukotrienes in the pathogenesis of aspirin-sensitive asthma that would be consistent with this theory, other evidence conflicts with it. An alternative theory proposes that the pathogenesis of reactions involves removal of prostanoid (prostaglandin) metabolites that regulate 5-lipoxygenase, with consequent upregulation of leukotriene production. Consistent with either theory, it has been found that patients with aspirin-sensitive asthma have higher urinary levels of leukotriene E4 (LTE4) after aspirin challenge compared with asthma patients without aspirin sensitivity. Aspirin-sensitive patients also have increased end-organ sensitivity to leukotrienes (e.g., enhanced bronchial reactivity to LTE4), which suggests that airway receptors are upregulated in aspirin-sensitive asthma. There is also evidence that aspirin reactions cause concomitant mast cell activation either by direct effects of aspirin and other NSAIDs on mast cells or by stimulation of mast cells by 5-lipoxygenase products.

Aspirin desensitization for patients with aspirin-induced bronchospasm is generally successful but must be performed with caution because of the frequent development of reactions during desensitization (Table 7.6). Although there have been reports of successful aspirin desensitization in patients who develop urticaria and angioedema from aspirin, efforts to desensitize such patients are often unsuccessful and significant adverse reactions can occur. Inhibition of 5-lipoxygenase by zileuton reduces urinary LTE4 levels and ablates respiratory and dermal reactions from aspirin. In most aspirin-sensitive patients, aspirin-induced bronchospasm can be blocked by leukotriene receptor antagonists (see Chapter 4).

Cytokines

Recombinant human cytokines, which are commonly used in the treatment of viral hepatitis and malignancies, can cause a variety of adverse reactions, some by novel mechanisms. Hypotension and a vascular leakage syndrome associated with IL-2 infusions have been correlated with activation of endothelial cells and of the classical complement cascade; a similar syndrome may occur with infusion of lymphokine-activated killer cells. Flu-like symptoms are commonly associated with interferon therapy. Macular, pruritic skin lesions with distinctive infiltrates characterized by lymphocytes, neutrophils, and eosinophils have been reported to develop at sites of subcutaneous injections of granulocyte–macrophage colony-stimulating factor.

Insulin

As a protein, insulin may cause a variety of immunologic reactions (all four types of Gell and Coombs reactions have been reported). In most patients, human insulin is less allergenic than porcine insulin (which is less aller-

Table 7.6 Aspirin Desensitization Protocol*

Time	Dose (mg)			
	Day 1	Day 2	Day 3	Day 4
8 AM	3	12	45	150
Noon	6	20	60	200
4 PM	12	30	100	325

* Incremental doses of powdered aspirin in gelatin capsules are given according to this schedule; if a fall in FEV_1 of 25% is achieved, bronchospasm should be treated and the provoking dose should be repeated every 3–24 h until no bronchospastic response occurs.

genic than bovine insulin), but in individual patients, porcine or bovine insulin may be the least allergenic. Some patients treated with nonhuman insulins have had systemic reactions to recombinant human insulin on first exposure.

More than 50% of patients who receive insulin develop antibodies against their insulin preparation after several weeks of administration. In many cases, patients develop IgE antibodies detectable by immediate-type skin testing and positive in vitro lymphocyte blastogenic responses to insulin, yet have no clinically apparent insulin allergy. To delay absorption and prolong activity, some insulin preparations contain protamine or zinc (e.g., in neutral protamine Hagedorn [NPH] or Lente insulins, respectively), which can cause allergic reactions. Patients who have received NPH insulins are at increased risk for anaphylaxis from protamine reversal of heparinization after cardiovascular surgery, although multiple mechanisms (only one being IgE) are probably responsible.

Local Insulin Allergy

Local reactions develop in approximately half of patients receiving insulin and typically appear within several weeks of the initiation of insulin therapy. Local reactions may occur within several days after resumption of insulin therapy after discontinuation of a previous course.

Immediate-type, IgE-mediated wheal and flare local reactions develop within 20 minutes after insulin injection. Although these often resolve within 1 hour, IgE-mediated, late-phase reactions may occur at 4 to 12 hours as part of a dual response. Isolated late responses may also occur from immune-complex–mediated Arthus reactions. Local reactions from delayed-type lymphocytic mechanisms (usually 24–72 h after injection) may also occur.

Usually, local reactions are minimal, do not require treatment, and resolve with continued insulin administration (possibly by action of anti-insulin IgG-blocking antibodies). More severe local reactions can be reduced with antihistamine administration or by dividing the insulin dose into injections at separate sites. Skin testing may identify other insulin preparations to which the patient is less sensitive. Local adverse effects may also be caused by intradermal rather than subcutaneous injection. Local reactions to the protamine component of NPH insulin may be avoided by switching to Lente insulin. Local reactions to zinc in insulin preparations have also been reported. Some patients tolerate regular insulin but cannot tolerate the usually more immunogenic Lente insulin.

Systemic Insulin Allergy
Generalized, immediate-type reactions (e.g., generalized urticaria, angioedema, and anaphylactic shock) are unusual. These IgE-mediated, systemic reactions almost always occur after reinstitution of insulin in patients sensitized by previous insulin administration and may be preceded by increasingly large local reactions.

Insulin therapy should not be interrupted if a systemic reaction to insulin occurs and continued insulin therapy is essential. Skin testing may identify an insulin preparation of lesser antigenicity. The next dose after the systemic reaction dose is usually reduced to one third of the dose that caused the reaction. Successive doses are gradually increased in two- to five-unit increments until the dose required for diabetic control is attained.

Insulin skin testing and desensitization are required when insulin treatment has been interrupted for more than 24 to 48 hours. Caution is required because of the risk of systemic reactions and hypoglycemia from insulin used in desensitization. Successful desensitization (Table 7.7) is associated with a decline in serum levels of IgE, skin test reactivity to insulin, and occasionally insulin resistance.

IgE-mediated anaphylaxis to protamine in NPH insulin has been reported and should be considered in the differential diagnosis of patients having reactions to NPH or protamine zinc insulin preparations. Intradermal skin tests showing higher reactivity to NPH insulin compared with regular insulin at the same concentration would support the diagnosis.

Insulin Resistance
Insulin resistance is defined as being present when (in the absence of ketoacidosis) more than 200 units of insulin per day for more than 2 days is required. Nonimmunologic insulin resistance may be associated with endocrinopathies, corticosteroid therapy, infections, and obesity. Immunologic insulin resistance most commonly occurs because patients develop high titers of circulating antibodies (predominantly IgG) to insulin. Usually it develops in patients over 40 years of age during their first year of insulin treatment and develops over several weeks, although the onset may be abrupt. A rare form of insulin resis-

Table 7.7 Insulin Desensitization Protocol

Day	Time	Route	Type	Units*
1	AM	ID	Reg	0.00001
1	Noon	ID	Reg	0.0001
1	PM	ID	Reg	0.001
2	AM	ID	Reg	0.01
2	Noon	ID	Reg	0.1
2	PM	ID	Reg	1.0
3	AM	ID	Reg	2.0
3	Noon	SQ	Reg	4.0
3	PM	SQ	Reg	8.0
4	AM	SQ	Reg	12.0
4	Noon	SQ	Reg	16.0
5	AM	SQ	NPH/Lente	20.0
6	AM	SQ	NPH/Lente	25.0
7	AM	SQ	NPH/Lente	Increase 5.0 U/d until therapeutic level is reached

ID = intradermal; NPH/Lente = long-acting insulin; Reg = regular crystalline zinc insulin; SQ = subcutaneous.
*The starting dose may be modified by the patient's insulin sensitivity, based on skin testing, 24–48 h after start of severe reaction.
Modified from Anderson JA, Adkinson NF Jr. Allergic reactions to drugs and biologic agents. JAMA. 1987;258:2891–9.

tance caused by circulating antibodies to tissue insulin receptors is associated with acanthosis nigricans and lipodystrophy. Coexistent insulin allergy may be present in up to one third of patients with insulin resistance.

Because high doses of insulin used during insulin resistance can saturate anti-insulin antibody and cause hypoglycemia, hospitalization and close monitoring of glucose levels are required during treatment for insulin resistance. Approximately half of patients benefit from substitution, with an insulin preparation found to be less reactive on skin testing. Corticosteroid therapy (e.g., prednisone 30–100 mg/d) benefits most patients within several days to weeks, although its mechanism of action is uncertain. When improvement occurs, corticosteroids may be tapered and administered using alternate-day dosing regimens.

Radiographic Contrast Media

Radiographic contrast media cause non–IgE-mediated anaphylactoid reactions that may involve direct mast cell and complement activation. Because allergic reactions to shellfish are IgE-mediated reactions to shellfish proteins and not to iodine, there is no significant association between shellfish allergy and radiographic contrast sensitivity. Because contrast-media reactions are not IgE-mediated, immediate-type skin testing is not predictive of reaction risk. Test dosing is not helpful in evaluation. Patients who have a history of an anaphylactoid reaction to radiographic contrast media at any time in the past (even if they have tolerated a subsequent administration of contrast media without incident) should be considered to be at significantly increased risk for a repeat anaphylactoid reaction. This risk can be reduced with use of newer nonionic contrast agents (although these are far more costly than standard contrast agents) and medication pretreatment. One commonly used regimen involves corticosteroids (e.g., prednisone 50 mg orally at 13 h, 7 h, and 1 h before contrast administration), antihistamines (e.g., diphenhydramine 50 mg orally at 1 h before administration), and oral adrenergic agents (e.g., ephedrine 25 mg or albuterol 4 mg orally at 1 h before administration). Regimens that administer corticosteroids only 1 to 2 hours before contrast administration are not recommended as efficacious in preventing reactions; therefore, patients should be informed that, despite precautions, a reaction may still occur.

Strategies for Prevention, Diagnosis, and Management of Drug Allergy

General considerations in the prevention, diagnosis, and management of drug allergy are summarized in Box 7.2. An assessment often must be made about the relative risks, potential benefits, and alternatives to administration of a drug suspected to pose a risk to a patient. Initial analysis requires review of the history and physical findings found at the time of a suspected adverse reaction. Tests to evaluate drug allergy are limited because of several factors. Many immunologic reactions are directed not against the drug itself but against drug metabolites. Small-molecular-weight drugs and metabolites may act as haptens that must be coupled to carrier proteins to be used in testing, and some of the immunologic mechanisms responsible for adverse reactions have not been well defined. Depending on the clinical setting, a variety of techniques and approaches may be applicable to the diagnosis and management of drug allergy. The following discussion of these techniques is intended to summarize their appropriate clinical applications and limitations and to provide examples (rather than a comprehensive discussion) about how to perform the techniques. Consultation with an experienced allergist–immunologist can provide additional assistance.

> **Box 7.2 General Considerations in Clinical Evaluation of Drug Reactions**
>
> Identify drugs that have a history of causing problems in an individual, determine whether there are cross-reacting agents, and avoid them.
>
> If a late reaction such as a drug rash occurs, take a careful history of all drugs used in the past month, because it is possible that the causative drug has been discontinued.
>
> Drugs administered with impunity for prolonged periods (e.g., months to years) are rarely responsible for adverse immunologic reactions. Consequently, when a reaction does occur, drugs introduced more recently are more likely to be responsible for the reaction.
>
> Have a high index of suspicion whenever adverse clinical manifestations develop in a patient, considering 1) that drug reactions can cause internal organ involvement (e.g., nephritis, hepatitis, isolated lymphadenopathy) and 2) that eosinophilia is often absent.
>
> If an immunologic drug reaction is suspected, stop all nonessential drugs and substitute non–cross-reactive drugs if possible.
>
> Modified from Dykewicz MS. Drug allergy. Compr Ther. 1997;22:353–9.

Strategies to Assess Risk and Reduce Drug Administration

Immediate-Type Skin Testing

This type of testing predicts IgE-mediated reactions only and cannot predict risk for non–IgE-mediated reactions, such as nonurticarial drug rashes. Immediate-type skin testing is currently limited to protein agents (e.g., heterologous antisera, insulin, chymopapain, streptokinase) or small-molecular-weight drugs whose allergenic metabolites have been identified and made available for skin testing (e.g., penicillin). Most nonpenicillin antibiotics (e.g., cephalosporins, sulfa) cannot be reliably skin tested, in part because all relevant allergenic metabolites are not identified or available for testing. In order to reduce the rare but possible risk of inducing a systemic reaction from immediate-type skin testing, skin testing should be performed by knowledgeable personnel, using appropriate dilutions of the drug to be tested. Solutions used for testing should be of concentrations that have been validated for specificity and sensitivity (i.e., dilute enough to be nonirritating and therefore not likely to cause nonspecific local irritant reactions but concentrated enough to afford a high degree of sensitivity). Intradermal testing should generally be preceded by epicutaneous (prick or scratch) testing, which has less risk for causing a systemic reaction. If epicutaneous tests are negative when assessed at 20 minutes, intradermal tests (which are more sensitive than epicutaneous tests) are then placed and subsequently read at 20 minutes. The drug solution must not be injected subcutaneously, because skin tests may then be falsely negative. Simultaneously, a positive histamine control skin test and a negative diluent control test are placed, because the results of the control sites must be compared with those of the drug skin tests. A negative response to a histamine control skin test suggests that the skin tests are being suppressed by medications such as H_1 (but not H_2) antihistamines, tricyclic antidepressants, and some phenothiazines. These agents must be withheld for at least several days (and in the case of astemizole, 4–6 wk) before skin testing. Contrary to common misconception, corticosteroid administration does not preclude performance of immediate-type skin testing, although steroids can impair delayed-type skin testing (e.g., PPD [purified protein derivative] testing).

In Vitro Testing

Available in vitro tests for specific IgE are less sensitive than skin tests for detecting specific IgE and, therefore, have limited use except when it is impossible to perform immediate skin tests (e.g., when interfering medications cannot be stopped). Immunologic hemolytic anemia is diagnosed by the indirect Coombs test and immune thrombocytopenia by complement fixation, agglutination reactions, and platelet lysis. The association between lymphocyte proliferative responses to drugs and nonurticarial drug rashes is fair for antiseizure medications but poor for sulfonamides; consequently, the use of such assays is investigational.

Approaches To Reduce the Risk of Immunologic Reactions from Drug Administration

Test Dosing

When the probability of true allergy is low, yet may exist in a patient, test dosing is used to administer a drug more safely, although reactions may still occur. First, the patient is given a drug in an initial dose that is below that which could cause serious reaction. This is followed by subsequent, large-increment dose increases up to full-dose therapy. Although this approach can be used for many drugs, it is not reliable for some agents (e.g., radiographic contrast media) that can cause reactions at full-dose therapy, even though lower doses administered during test dosing were well tolerated.

Desensitization

Desensitization is a general term that may pertain to several techniques that are applied in different clinical settings when the probability of drug allergy is high but drug administration is essential (e.g., insulin in uncontrolled diabetes, penicillin in neurosyphilis). Compared with test dosing, incremental dose increases generally are much smaller. If desensitization for an antibiotic is being considered, it may be appropriate to obtain consultation from an infectious disease specialist to document need for the drug. Because of the risk of adverse reactions during desensitization, only physicians who are aware of the risks, limitations, and precautions required for desensitization should perform it.

Desensitization by oral administration has less risk for anaphylaxis than parenteral administration and therefore is preferred by some authorities. Others prefer parenteral administration because gastrointestinal absorption may be impaired (e.g., in cystic fibrosis or diabetic gastroparesis), requiring greater intervals between doses to assure that there is no reaction before administration of the next dose.

Once desensitization has been achieved, drug administration must be continued or desensitization may be lost. If a drug is discontinued after desensitization, the patient will likely need to be desensitized again before readministration.

Desensitization When There Is High Risk for an IgE-Mediated Reaction
In this setting, the principle is to cause controlled, subclinical anaphylaxis. Desensitization begins with a very small initial dose of the drug that would not cause serious reaction (e.g., one millionth of full dose), with subsequent small dose increases (in contrast to test dosing) to reach full dose (*see* Tables 7.3 and 7.4). Depending on circumstances, this can usually be done within 24 hours, although it may be preferable to perform desensitization over several days. It generally is advisable to desensitize in a monitored setting if there is significant risk for a life-threatening reaction. If a reaction occurs during desensitization, the reaction is treated, the last dose tolerated is repeated, and further dose increases are made more slowly. Mild reactions during desensitization are not unusual.

Desensitization When There Is High Risk for Non–IgE-Mediated Immediate Reaction
Depending on the agent and the type of allergic reaction caused by the drug, desensitization may or may not be possible. For example, patients having only

respiratory symptoms (e.g., bronchospasm) from aspirin or NSAIDs can often be desensitized successfully over 4 to 5 days (although mild reactions are frequent) by giving three to four doses of increasing amounts of drug each day and by monitoring for decreases in spirometry after each dose (*see* Table 7.6). However, patients having cutaneous reactions from aspirin (e.g., urticaria, angioedema) are very difficult to desensitize. It may not be possible to desensitize patients to narcotics because of the direct effects of these drugs on mast cell–mediator release. Desensitization to prevent anaphylactoid reactions to radiographic contrast media is not effective.

Desensitization for Late Reactions (Nonurticarial Rashes)

Very slow desensitization (with gradual administration of drug in increasing amounts over days to weeks) may permit tolerance to a drug that has caused nonurticarial skin rashes. Desensitization to sulfasalazine (in those who have developed late skin rashes to its sulfa moiety) generally can be performed successfully by using a 1-month-long protocol (*see* Table 7.5). This, however, requires monitoring of blood counts and blood chemistries to assure that adverse internal organ reactions are not developing, and the process should be supervised by a physician experienced in this approach. Although there is little literature about this type of desensitization to other agents, this process may be considered in unusual circumstances in which there are no good therapeutic alternatives. Attempts to desensitize more rapidly (over 1–2 d) to drugs causing nonurticarial reactions is more likely to fail but can be successful.

Premedication

In limited circumstances when an anaphylactoid reaction is of concern, pretreatment of the patient with corticosteroids, antihistamines, and oral adrenergic agents may reduce the risk for a reaction. (*See* Radiographic Contrast Media.) This approach is generally not reliable for preventing IgE-mediated anaphylaxis.

"Treating Through"

In extreme circumstances when continued administration of a drug is essential but is causing a reaction such as a late drug rash or interstitial nephritis, continued drug administration may be tolerated if corticosteroids and antihistamines are given to suppress the immunologic reaction. Risks of this approach are that a skin rash may progress to exfoliation or to Stevens–Johnson syndrome or that patients may develop internal organ involvement, including nephritis, hepatitis, or a serum sickness–like syndrome. Careful monitoring of patient status is essential.

Treatment

Treatment of Acute Adverse Immunologic Drug Reactions

In these circumstances, all suspect drugs that are nonessential should be stopped, and any new drugs added to a patient's treatment regimen should not have cross-reactivity with incriminated drugs.

Treatment of Immediate Reactions

Epinephrine, antihistamines, and in some settings, corticosteroids and other resuscitative measures are indicated for treatment of anaphylaxis (*see* Chapter 6).

Treatment of Late Reactions (Drug Rashes, Serum Sickness)

For very mild maculopapular rashes, antihistamines alone may be adequate. For more severe rashes, rashes that are progressing, or rashes associated with constitutional symptoms (e.g., fever, nausea, arthralgias) corticosteroids should be added to treatment. An initial recommended dose is prednisone, at least 40 to 60 mg/d (1–2 mg/kg/d in children), with tapering once the reaction has stabilized. For prolonged, severe reactions, several weeks of prednisone may be required, but it is often possible to convert prednisone administration to an alternate-day morning regimen after 1 week of treatment.

SUGGESTED READINGS

Anderson JA. Allergic reactions to drugs and biologic agents. JAMA. 1992;286:2845–58.

Anderson JA, Adkinson NF Jr. Allergic reactions to drugs and biologic agents. JAMA. 1987;258:2891–9.

Anne S, Reisman RE. Risk of administering cephalosporin antibiotics to patients with histories of penicillin allergy. Ann Allergy Asthma Immunol. 1995;74:167–70.

DeShazo R, Nelson H. An approach to the patient with a history of local anesthetic hypersensitivity: experience with 90 patients. J Allergy Clin Immunol. 1982;69:275–82.

DeSwarte RD. Drug allergy. In: Patterson R., ed. Allergic Diseases: Diagnosis and Management. 5th ed. Philadelphia: JB Lippincott; 1997:317–412.

Gadde J, Spence M, Wheeler B, Adkinson NF Jr. Clinical experience with penicillin skin testing in a large inner-city STD clinic. JAMA. 1993;270:2456–63.

Lee TH. Mechanism of bronchospasm in aspirin-sensitive asthma [Editorial]. Am Rev Respir Dis. 1993;148:1442–3.

Moss RB, Babin S, Hsu Y-P, et al. Allergy to semisynthetic penicillins in cystic fibrosis. J Pediatr. 1984;104:460–6.

Parker PJ, Parrinello JT, Condemi JJ, Rosenfeld SI. Penicillin resensitization among hospitalized patients. J Allergy Clin Immunol. 1991;88:213–7.

Polk RE. Anaphylactoid reactions to glycoprotein antibiotics. J Antimicrobial Ther. 1991;27(Suppl B):17–29.

Purdy BH, Philips DM, Summers RW. Desensitization for sulfasalazine skin rash. Ann Int Med. 1984;100:512–4.

Saxon A, Adelman DC, Patel A, et al. Imipenem cross-reactivity with penicillin in humans. J Allergy Clin Immunol. 1986;82:213–7.

Saxon A, Swabb EA, Adkinson NF Jr. Investigation into the immunologic cross-reactivity of aztreonam with other beta-lactam antibiotics. Am J Med. 1985;78(Suppl A):19–26.

Simon SR, Black HR, Moser M, Berland WE. Cough and ACE inhibitors. Arch Int Med. 1992;152:1698–700.

Sogn DD, Evans R III, Shepherd GM, et al. Results of the National Institute of Allergy and Infectious Diseases collaborative clinical trial to test the predictive value of skin testing with major and minor penicillin determinant derivatives in hospitalized patients. Arch Int Med. 1992;152:1025–32.

Sullivan T, Yecies L, Shatz G, et al. Desensitization of patients allergic to penicillin using orally administered beta-lactam antibodies. J Allergy Clin Immunol. 1982;69:275–8.

Wickern GM, Nish WA, Bitner AS, Freeman TM. Allergy to beta-lactams: a survey of current practices. J Allergy Clin Immunol. 1994;94:725–31.

Chapter 8

Immunologic Lung Diseases

Jordan N. Fink, MD
Michael C. Zacharisen, MD

Although IgE–mast cell–mediated inflammation that results in asthma is the most common immunologic lung disease, other immunologic mechanisms may induce other types of allergic lung diseases. Allergic bronchopulmonary aspergillosis (ABPA) is due to a marked inflammatory reaction to *Aspergillus* in the airway, resulting in airway destruction and parenchymal inflammation. Hypersensitivity pneumonitis (HP) is associated with sensitization and repeated exposure to any of a variety of organic dusts that induce pulmonary infiltrative and granulomatous disease, with systemic features likely on a T-cell–mediated immune process. This chapter discusses these two disorders.

Allergic Bronchopulmonary Aspergillosis

Aspergillus is a ubiquitous organism that has been associated with a number of syndromes, ranging from asthma in the atopic individual to invasive systemic disease in the immunocompromised host. *Aspergillus* may colonize pre-existing cavitary pulmonary disease, resulting in a fungus ball or aspergilloma and can complicate allergic asthma or cystic fibrosis by manifesting as ABPA. Cases of ABPA have been recognized since the first clinical description was reported in England in 1952 and in the United States in 1969.

Allergic bronchopulmonary aspergillosis is an immunologic pulmonary inflammatory mediated by immune process and can cause complications in patients with

161

asthma and cystic fibrosis, who have an increased prevalence of ABPA (1). The organism responsible for ABPA is usually *Aspergillus fumigatus*, which colonizes damaged airways, causing characteristic clinical, immunologic, radiographic, and pathologic features that vary from mild bronchospasm to fibrotic parenchymal disease (2). Progression to end-stage pulmonary fibrosis may occur if ABPA is not recognized early. Effective treatment is directly related to early recognition and the institution of anti-inflammatory rather than antifungal therapy.

Case 8.1

A 35-year-old white male landscaper with moderate asthma for 12 years presented as a new patient after a recent hospitalization for asthma exacerbation and "pneumonia." Although his asthma symptoms had been moderately well controlled, he had over the preceding 2 years several flares of bronchitis with dark mucus production and more-difficult-to-control asthma that required higher doses of inhaled corticosteroids. On several occasions he sought treatment at urgent care centers and received bursts of oral corticosteroids, with initial rapid relief of symptoms. Previous chest radiographs were not available, but pneumonia was diagnosed twice previously. He had just completed a 7-day course of prednisone. He had a history of mild allergic rhinitis. Tobacco history was 10 pack-years. Family history was significant, for his brother has asthma.

Examination revealed normal head and neck, with mild expiratory wheezing on forced expiration without crackles. He exhibited a deep, moist cough but was unable to expectorate sputum. There was no clubbing, cyanosis, or edema. Office spirometry was consistent with mild obstruction partially reversible with β-2-agonist bronchodilators.

Skin testing was positive to multiple allergens, including animal dander, dust mite, and various molds (*Alternaria*, *Cladosporium*, and *Aspergillus*). The total IgE level was elevated at 7000 ng/mL, and eosinophilia was absent.

The patient was diagnosed with allergic asthma and prescribed high doses of inhaled corticosteroids and a long-acting inhaled bronchodilator. He was discharged with a peak flow meter and holding chamber for his metered-dose inhaler.

An urgent follow-up visit 4 weeks later for an asthma exacerbation revealed moderate dyspnea, productive cough of dark plugs, and low-grade fever. Serum was obtained, a precipitin to *Aspergillus fumigatus* was demonstrated, and elevated titers of IgG- and IgE-specific antibody were documented. The total IgE level was 17,000 ng/mL, and chest radiograph revealed patchy infiltrates and atelectasis, primarily in the upper lobes. Sputum smear revealed fungal elements, and culture grew *Aspergillus* species. A diagnosis of ABPA was made, and prednisone therapy was initiated at 60 mg/d for 3 weeks, then slowly decreased to 20 mg every other day. Follow-up chest radiograph revealed infiltrate resolution and an IgE level of 500 ng/mL. Symptoms were also significantly improved. Chest computed tomography (CT) was normal, without evidence of central bronchiectasis.

Clinical Features

The major clinical features of ABPA include 1) asthma, 2) recurrent pulmonary infiltrates, 3) immediate wheal-and-flare skin reactivity and serum-precipitating antibodies to *A. fumigatus*, 4) elevated total serum IgE levels, 5) peripheral blood eosinophilia, 6) elevated levels of *Aspergillus*-specific serum IgE and IgG (when compared with levels from *Aspergillus*-sensitive asthmatics), and 7) central bronchiectasis with normal distal structures (1) (Box 8.1). Additional features include a late inflammatory skin-test response (following the immediate wheal-and-flare reaction induced by an extract of the organism *A. fumigatus*), positive culture of *A. fumigatus* in the sputum, and the expectoration of brown mucus plugs containing the organism. All features may not be present in each patient with ABPA. The treatment of asthma with corticosteroids may reduce the eosinophilia, elevated total serum IgE levels, *Aspergillus*-specific IgE levels and precipitating antibodies. Early in the disease, bronchiectasis may not be evident.

The diagnosis of ABPA should be considered in patients of all ages who have asthma (*see* Box 8.1). ABPA has been described in young children, adolescents, and adults. The symptoms present usually as episodic cough, purulent sputum with sputum plugs, dyspnea, wheezing, fever, chills, and malaise. Hemoptysis may be scant or prominent. Because there is progression, features of fibrotic lung disease with cough and dyspnea may predominate. The physical examination may be normal or show features ranging from pneumonitis with consolidation, asthma with wheezing, or bronchiectasis with dry or moist rales. In end-stage disease, nail clubbing, cyanosis, tachypnea, and features of cor pulmonale may be found (2).

The clinical laboratory findings include an immediate wheal-and-flare skin-prick reaction to an extract of *A. fumigatus* and, in one third of patients, a late-onset skin response of erythema and induration following the immediate wheal-and-flare reaction (Fig. 8.1). Thus, the absence of an immediate wheal-and-flare reaction to *Aspergillus* almost always rules out ABPA. If sputum production occurs, it may contain eosinophils and Charcot–Leyden crystals. *Aspergillus* species may be found in sputum cultures in approximately 60% of

---

Box 8.1 Characteristics of Allergic Bronchopulmonary Aspergillosis

Asthma, usually allergic	Elevated total serum IgE levels
Recurrent pulmonary infiltrates	Blood eosinophilia
IgE skin reactivity to *Aspergillus*	Elevated *Aspergillus*-specific IgG and IgE
Precipitating antibodies to *Aspergillus*	Central bronchiectasis

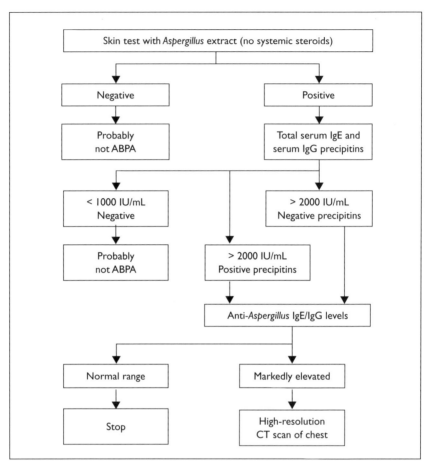

Figure 8.1 Clinical evaluation for allergic bronchopulmonary aspergillosis (ABPA). CT = computed tomography; IgE = immunoglobulin E; IgG = immunoglobulin G. (Adapted from Slavin RG. Allergic Bronchopulmonary Aspergillosis in Atlas of Allergies. 2nd ed. St. Louis, MO: Mosby-Wolfe; 1996.)

patients. Peripheral blood eosinophilia ranging from 1000 to 3000/mm^3 may be prominent unless corticosteroids are being used as treatment.

Immunologic Diagnosis

Serologic studies are often helpful in the diagnosis of ABPA (3). Total serum IgE levels are usually over 1000 ng/mL in patients not on corticosteroids, but in some cases a marked elevation of IgE level up to 120,000 ng/mL or more may be detected. The total serum IgE levels decrease within several months of corticosteroid treatment, but in controlled ABPA the baseline IgE level may still be elevated above normal.

The evaluation of *Aspergillus*-specific serum IgE and IgG levels may also be helpful, because patients with ABPA have several-fold elevations of specific antibody when compared with *Aspergillus*-sensitive asthmatics with no clinical features of ABPA. Precipitating antibodies can be demonstrated by gel immunodiffusion in up to 90% of affected patients. Again, corticosteroids may reduce or eliminate this serologic reaction.

The diagnosis of ABPA is thus solidified by detecting IgE and IgG antibodies to the organism. This requires the use of reliable antigen and sensitive immunologic techniques. Currently, there are no standardized antigens available for skin or in vitro testing; therefore, commercial or "home-grown" antigens are used. In recent years, purified antigens have been isolated, and they may enhance our immunodiagnostic capabilities in the future.

Current techniques useful in the diagnosis include gel immunodiffusion (for determination of IgG-precipitating antibodies) and enzyme-linked immunosorbent assay or radioallergosorbent test (for detection and semiquantitation of specific IgE and IgG antibodies) (4). Demonstration of precipitins via gel diffusion is almost universal in ABPA, and the detection of levels of specific IgE and IgG greater than twice those of patients with *Aspergillus*-induced asthma is significant in asthma patients who have not been treated with steroids. Determinations of total serum IgE level are useful in the diagnosis and in following the patient's response to treatment as well as predicting exacerbations.

Laboratory Features

Pulmonary function often demonstrates features of asthma, with reduction in air flow and persistent obstruction. Restrictive features with decreased lung volumes may be found in end-stage disease. Most importantly, early intervention and treatment with corticosteroids has been reported to prevent deterioration of pulmonary function. It should be noted that normal pulmonary function does not rule out ABPA if the patient is evaluated during remission. Radiographic features may be helpful in the diagnosis of ABPA (5). Standard chest radiographs or tomographic scans have been of value, but thin-section CT of the hilar and perihilar areas has been an important diagnostic adjunct and should be carried out in all suspected patients, because central bronchiectasis can be demonstrated in most patients with ABPA (6). The CT chest scan also provides baseline evaluation of the bronchial tree, which can then be used to gauge response. It is important to recognize that detectable bronchial changes are not present in all patients with ABPA. In these patients, early treatment of their ABPA may prevent further progression (7).

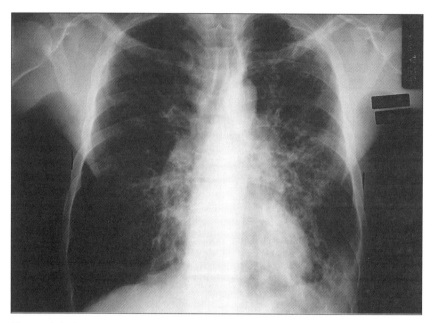

Figure 8.2 Chest radiograph of patient with allergic bronchopulmonary aspergillosis. Perihilar and left lower lobe infiltrates are evident.

Standard chest radiographs demonstrate transient infiltrates and mucoid impaction in ABPA (Fig. 8.2). Proximal bronchiectasis is characteristic; bullae and pneumothorax may occur with pulmonary fibrosis in advanced disease. Bronchiectasis or ectatic bronchi with edema of the airway wall present as ring shadows or parallel-line, "tram-line" shadows. Infiltrates may present as dense consolidation or as nodules in upper or lower lobes. Mucoid impaction presents in dilated bronchi as "toothpaste" shadows and are called "gloved-finger" shadows when the bronchi are filled with secretions.

Bronchiectasis is represented as central dilation and distal tapering and can be seen in ABPA and cystic fibrosis but not in postinfection bronchiectasis. Thin-section CT provides significant detail of the proximal structures and dilated bronchi (Fig. 8.3).

Pathology

The patient with ABPA usually does not need lung biopsy for diagnosis because of the characteristic clinical features. Examination of lung tissue from ABPA patients has shown nonspecific features that vary in the same biopsy. The lesions have features of mucoid impaction, pulmonary fibrosis, eosinophilic pneumonia, granulomas, obliterative bronchiolitis, and cystic fi-

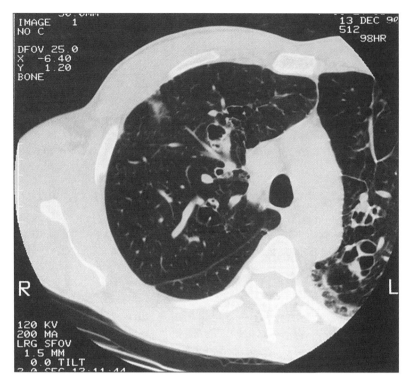

Figure 8.3 Computed tomography of the chest in a patient with allergic bronchopulmonary aspergillosis. Marked interstitial infiltrates and ectatic bronchi are evident.

brosis. Fungi may be detected within bronchi surrounded by eosinophils. Invasion of pulmonary parenchyma is rare. Collagen replacement of submucosal glands and smooth muscle may be present. Mucoid impaction presents with bronchial lumens filled with concentric layers of epithelial cells, basophils, eosinophils, and debris. The bronchi may be similar to asthma, with thickening of the basement membrane; smooth muscle hypertrophy; hyperplasia of mucus glands; and infiltration with eosinophils, plasma cells, and lymphocytes.

Stages

Allergic bronchopulmonary aspergillosis has been classified into five clinical stages, ranging from the acute to fibrosis. Patients may progress from one stage to another (8).

Acute Stage
The acute stage is the early phase of ABPA, with minimal to classic clinical features and rapid response to prednisone.

Remission Stage
Remission may then occur with absence of symptoms and stability of the underlying asthma; corticosteroids may then be discontinued. The total serum IgE level remains low. This stage may last a variable period or become permanent.

Recurrence Stage
The third stage of ABPA begins with recurrence of the acute phase and is often preceded by at least a twofold rise in total serum IgE level. Classic findings of the disease are present, and the response to corticosteroids is as rapid as before.

Dependent Stage
The patient may then develop corticosteroid-dependent asthma. This is likely related to the severity of the underlying inflammatory process and is the most common presentation of the disease. Appropriate therapy of patients in this stage can induce stabilization without progression.

Fibrosis Stage
The final stage of ABPA is fibrotic lung disease. Bronchiectasis is prominent and *Aspergillus* or *Pseudomonas* may be found in the respiratory tree. Pulmonary fibrosis progresses and fatalities occur. Early treatment appears to prevent progression of ABPA to fibrosis.

Differential Diagnosis

Allergic bronchopulmonary aspergillosis has features of eosinophilic blood and lung diseases, pulmonary infiltration, and bronchiectasis. Its presentation is modified by previous anti-asthma therapy, especially oral corticosteroids. Consequently, both eosinophilia and serum IgE levels may be low in patients so treated. Asthma without ABPA may also present with eosinophilia, whereas chronic eosinophilic pneumonia has a "ground-glass" appearance, unlike the infiltrates of ABPA.

Other pulmonary infiltrative diseases (e.g., vasculitis, Churg–Strauss syndrome, leukemia, lymphoma, and Wegener's granulomatosis) may be considered. Serologic tests and chest tomographic scans should clarify the diagnosis. Elevation in sweat chloride levels points to the diagnosis of cystic fibrosis, but aspergillosis as a complication of that disease must also be considered (9).

Pathogenesis

Aspergillus, particularly *A. fumigatus*, is widely distributed in nature, and because of its ubiquitous nature, practically all individuals may demonstrate low levels of antifungal antibodies. Normal defense mechanisms usually protect the individual from adverse responses; however, some individuals with atopy may develop ABPA on exposure to *A. fumigatus*. The immune mechanism(s) involved in ABPA are not completely understood; both humoral- and cell-mediated immune responses have been implicated.

Continuous exposure to *Aspergillus* through the inhalation of spores that colonize the respiratory tract may induce a prolonged inflammatory response with eosinophilic infiltration and mast cell accumulation, which may release pro-inflammatory cytokines in response to *Aspergillus* allergens combining with specific IgE. This inflammation leads to chemotaxis of additional eosinophils and inflammatory cells and to the activation of T cells and macrophages, which may begin a granulomatous process in the lung seen in some patients with ABPA. Anti-*Aspergillus* antibody enables *Aspergillus* antigen and mycelial fragments to penetrate and deposit in the lung parenchyma. Eosinophils are a source of sulfidopeptide leukotrienes, which then promote mucus production, bronchoconstriction, hyperemia, and edema.

The lung lesions are bronchocentric rather than angiocentric, and the lack of vasculitis or deposition of complement and immunoglobulin in the vessel walls suggests that immune complexes do not mediate the lesions. Specific IgE can be detected in the germinal centers of pulmonary lymph nodes, and IgG can be detected in the lung parenchyma. *Aspergillus* hyphae frequently have been demonstrated by silver staining in the lungs of patients. *Aspergillus*-specific IgG, IgA, and IgE antibodies are elevated in ABPA, and enhanced total IgE levels and pulmonary peripheral blood eosinophilia appear to be the result of fungal colonization.

Cell-mediated immune responses appear to be important in patients with ABPA (10). The enhanced IgE synthesis and eosinophil proliferation and activation are both regulated by T cells. T-helper-inducer cells show a moderate increase in the peripheral blood mononuclear cells (PBMC) when compared with lung lavage cells. Suppresser cells are slightly enhanced in ABPA with cystic fibrosis and in vitro antigen-induced proliferation of PBMC is also vigorous in these patients. Active in vitro IgE production in PBMC cultures stimulated with *Aspergillus* antigen has been reported in ABPA, and the B cells of patients with ABPA and ABPA with cystic fibrosis have been shown to spontaneously secrete IgE (11). Culture supernatants from *Aspergillus*-stimulated T cells enhance the IgE synthesis by B cells, which suggests that *Aspergillus* itself may have immunoregulatory features. In addition, recent reports indicate the production of both B-cell activating and suppressive factors, which regulate IgE production and T- and B-cell interactions.

T lymphocytes regulate B-cell IgE synthesis and eosinophil differentiation and activation. In ABPA CD4+ Th2 cells secrete cytokines, such as interleukin (IL)-4, that enhance IgE synthesis by B cells and stimulate production and secretion of eosinophil growth and activation factor (IL-5). Eosinophils are increased in the circulation and the lungs of patients with ABPA. Evidence indicates that eosinophils are major inflammatory cells in asthma and allergy. Major basic protein, which is a constituent of the eosinophil granule, is implicated in the epithelial shedding and mast cell degranulation within the airway. Other proteins associated with eosinophil granules (e.g., eosinophil cationic protein, eosinophil-derived neurotoxins, and eosinophil peroxidase) may also be inflammatory. Recent evidence suggests that *Aspergillus* antigens may induce T cells to secrete mediators that enhance eosinophilic activity.

Animal models of ABPA provide insight into the pathogenesis of the disease. Mice exposed by injection or inhalation to *Aspergillus* spores developed elevated specific IgE and eosinophils, which are under cytokine control and enhance total IgE production (either directly or indirectly) through activation of the Th2 pathway.

Features of ABPA may be found in other allergic bronchopulmonary mycoses related to colonization by *Helminthosporium, Curvularia, Candida, Drechslera, Stemphyllium,* and *Penicillium.* Appropriate bronchial culture and serologic studies are of value in these cases. ABPA should be considered as complications in other specific disorders. Up to 15% of patients with cystic fibrosis may develop ABPA, with clinical and immunologic abnormalities identical to those of patients with ABPA without cystic fibrosis. The diagnosis may be particularly difficult, because the cystic fibrotic patient has a relatively higher prevalence of atopy, colonization, and immune responses to *Aspergillus.* Also, chest radiographic features are similar to those of ABPA. Serum IgE elevation and the demonstration of high levels of *Aspergillus*-specific IgE may be clues in the diagnosis (9).

Allergic bronchopulmonary aspergillosis also has been associated with environmental exposures from hay or compost; it also appears in those individuals using contaminated marijuana.

Treatment

The goals of treatment in ABPA are to control the asthma and to prevent exacerbations of ABPA in order to keep the patient stabilized. Asthma should be controlled with pharmacotherapy and, when indicated, environmental control and immunotherapy. Immunotherapy, however, should not include *Aspergillus* antigens because of the risk of immune complex disease, with interaction of antigen with specific serum IgG antibodies.

The infiltrates of ABPA may not always be symptomatic. Therefore, it is important to follow patients at intervals, with the determination of total serum

IgE levels, because a significant increase is often predictive of a flare of ABPA (12). Treatment should then be vigorously instituted. Although flares of ABPA may be asymptomatic, the onset of wheezing, sputum, fever, and systemic symptoms in stable asthma should be evaluated with a total serum IgE level and institution of appropriate therapy.

The pharmacotherapy of ABPA includes anti-asthma management and corticosteroids. Antifungal agents (e.g., amphotericin-B, clotrimazole, ketoconazole, itraconazole, and nystatin) have been tried, but corticosteroids remain the most effective agents. Inhaled anti-inflammatory agents (e.g., cromolyn, beclomethasone, flunisolide, or triamcinolone) do not consistently prevent recurrences of ABPA. During the acute flare of ABPA, prednisone should be administered at a dose of 0.5 mg/kg/d for several weeks until symptomatic improvement occurs and the pulmonary infiltrates resolve. The dose should then be converted to an alternate-day dose for up to 3 months. During this period, total serum IgE levels should decrease to less than or equal to 35% of pretreatment levels. The levels usually do not return to normal but rather approach baseline because levels of total serum IgE in patients with asymptomatic ABPA may be elevated.

The prednisone is tapered slowly and may eventually be discontinued in some patients. All patients need monitoring at intervals for potential exacerbations. Although repeated courses of corticosteroids may be needed with frequent recurrences, continuous corticosteroids may be instituted. Patients with end-stage disease may need prolonged corticosteroid therapy to maintain their remaining pulmonary integrity.

Hypersensitivity Pneumonitis

Immunologic respiratory diseases that involve immune mechanisms other than the inflammation induced by antigen-IgE–mast-cell–mediator release system may be the result of inhalation of antigens present in the susceptible individual's environment. There is an increasing awareness that a wide variety of inhaled biologic dusts, low-molecular-weight chemicals, and medications may induce disease of the pulmonary interstitium, alveoli, and the middle and terminal airways. The terms *hypersensitivity pneumonitis* (HP) and *extrinsic allergic alveolitis* have been used to describe this syndrome. It may occur in several forms, depending on the duration and amount of exposure to the offending agent, the nature of the agent, and the immunologic response of the patient (13). Although both asthma and HP result from immunologically induced inflammation, there are distinct clinical and immune-response differences between the two.

Case 8.2

A 49-year-old white male attorney returned to your office after 4 weeks of symptoms. He initially experienced chills, fever, cough, and a heavy feeling in his chest, beginning 8 weeks after moving into a newly renovated office in the courthouse building. His symptoms occurred after each work day and were relieved at home. He developed increasing malaise and cough over 3 weeks. A prescription for antitussives and penicillin was of no benefit. He continued to work and developed progressive dyspnea on exertion and chest tightness. His symptoms improved near the end of a 1-week vacation but then recurred by midday on his first day back to work. He returned to your office with mild dyspnea, temperature 38.7°C, pulse 110, respirations 24, and coughing.

Chest examination revealed dry crackles bilaterally. Spirometry reveal a forced vital capacity (FVC) of 75% and a forced expiratory volume after 1 second (FEV$_1$) of 70%. Chest radiograph revealed interstitial infiltrates.

Complete blood count revealed elevated leukocyte count of 18,000/mm^3.

A diagnosis of acute atypical pneumonia was made.

Macrolide antibiotics were started. He went back to work feeling well after 2 days of bed rest. Within 1 day, he again presents to your office with similar clinical findings, including the persistent infiltrate on chest radiograph. Spirometry again suggested a restrictive pattern and pulse oximetry was 85% on room air. He was admitted to the hospital with a Po$_2$ of 54 mm Hg; within 24 hours of initiating intravenous antibiotics and prednisone, the chest radiograph was normal and he was asymptomatic.

An industrial hygienist inspected the building and cultured bacteria from stagnant water found in the air-conditioning unit. Serum-precipitating antibodies were demonstrated in agar-gel diffusion techniques. The diagnosis of ventilation pneumonitis was made, and alterations in the cooling system were undertaken. The patient was able to return to work, developed no symptoms, and continued to have normal lung function.

Causative Agents

The antigens capable of inducing HP are numerous and may be derived from microorganisms (e.g., *Actinomycete* species, bacteria, fungi, amoebae), animal (e.g., avian and rodent species) and plant products, low-molecular-weight chemicals, and various pharmaceuticals (Table 8.1). Sensitization may occur via immune responses within the bronchial-associated lymphoid tissue or via recruitment of immunoreactive cells into the lung by cytokine release. Reactions are likely induced by antigens of 5 μm and smaller that can enter the

Table 8.1 Some Antigens That Cause Hypersensitivity Pneumonitis

Disease	Antigen	Source
Bacteria		
"Farmer's lung"	Thermophilic *Actinomycete* species	Moldy hay, compost, grain
Bagassosis	Thermophilic *Sacchari* species	Moldy sugarcane
Ventilation pneumonitis	Thermophilic *Candida* species, *Klebsiella* species	Humidifier/air-conditioner
"Mushroom-worker's lung"	Thermophilic *Viridis* species	Mushroom compost
Fungi		
"Malt-worker's lung"	*Aspergillus* species	Moldy malt dust
"Wood-worker's lung"	*Alternaria* species	Moldy wood dust
"Cheese-worker's lung"	*Penicilliium caseii*	Cheese mold
"Maple-bark–stripper's" disease	*Cryptostroma corticale*	Moldy maple bark
Suberosis	*Penicillium frequentans*	Moldy cork dust
Sequoiosis	*Pullularia* species	Moldy redwood dust
Summer type	*Trichosporum cutaneum*	Japanese house mold
"Machine-operator's lung"	*Pseudomonas fluorescens, Acinetobacter lwoffi*	Used metal-working fluid
Animal proteins		
"Bird-breeder's" disease	Avian serum proteins (pigeon, duck, turkey, lovebird)	Avian dust
"Pituitary-snuff–user's lung"	Bovine or porcine proteins	Pituitary snuff
"Laboratory-worker's lung"	Rat urine protein	Rat urine in dust
"Oyster-shell lung"	Oyster- or mollusk-shell protein	Shell dust
Insect proteins		
"Wheat-weevil" disease	*Sitophilus granarius*	Infested wheat flour
"Sericulturist's lung"	Silkworm larvae	Cocoon fluff
Amoebae		
Ventilation pneumonitis	*Naegleria gruberi, Acanthamoeba castellani*	Contaminated humidifier
Drugs		
Medication-induced disease	Amiodarone, gold, β-blockers, sulfonamides, bacille Calmette-Guérin, nitrofurantoin, minocycline, procarbazine, methotrexate	Drug
Chemicals		
"Paint-refinisher's" disease	Toluene diisocyanate	Paint catalyst
"Bathtub-refinisher's lung"	Diphenylmethane diisocyanate	Paint catalyst
"Epoxy-resin–worker's lung"	Phthalic anhydride	Epoxy resin
"Plastic-worker's lung"	Trimellitic anhydride	Plastics industry

alveoli. The absorption of soluble antigens from deposited organisms may also be important in the production of immunologic parenchymal disease. The inhaled organic dusts may have a variety of biologic effects (e.g., stimulation of alveolar macrophages, direct activation of the alternative pathway of complement, function as immunologic adjuvants) and often contain endotoxins or toxic substances that have enzymatic activity.

The most frequent antigens involved in HP are the thermophilic *Actinomycete* organisms that cause "farmer's lung." These organisms are ubiquitous and have been isolated from soil, manure, grain, compost, hay, and forced-air heating, cooling, and humidification systems. They are present in vegetable composts, mushroom piles, and in ventilation systems (14). Frequently, the antigen load may be heavy, particularly in the farming environment in which moldy hay can produce an estimated 750,000 *Actinomycete* spores per minute in the air.

Moldy hay is only one of numerous sources of thermophilic *Actinomycete* organisms on a dairy farm. The top layer of hay in silos provides a suitable environment for their growth. Emptying a silo often provokes an acute episode of "farmer's lung." Other sources of antigen include 1) piles of straw, cornstalks, sawdust, and other waste material used for bedding in the dairy barn; and 2) damp moldy oats, corn fodder, and any organic material that has molded and then warmed up to 50° to 60°C. Acute episodes occur most often in the late winter when the farmer, after having used up his supply of good fodder or bedding, piles up the moldy materials. In the barn, which is closed tight against the cold, he cannot avoid breathing clouds of spores, which may then induce disease.

Other common organisms involved in HP include fungi (e.g., *Alternaria, Penicillium,* and *Aspergillus*) present in certain occupational environments, such as soy sauce brewing, fishing-store workers handling moldy bait, farmers working in poorly constructed greenhouses, or workers removing and mending moldy wooden floors. Suberosis has been described in the cork industry, and sequoiosis has been found in the redwood lumber industry. "Cheeseworker's lung" is related to the inhalation of *Penicillium* spores, whereas "machine-operator's lung" is associated with *Pseudomonas*-contaminated metalworking fluids.

Spray air-conditioning systems have been implicated in several outbreaks of HP. In these systems, refrigerated water is sprayed into a chamber in which moving air is cooled. Contaminants of the system circulate in the air and are inhaled by employees of the office or factory, resulting in disease. Stagnant water and debris along with a furnace plenum (bonnet) temperature of 60°C are common to implicated systems. These features provide a milieu for the growth and proliferation of thermophilic *Actinomycete* organisms. Room humidifier and home ultrasonic humidifiers that generate aerosolized water droplets in the range of 0.5 to 3.0 μm have also been implicated, although the organisms in these cases may not necessarily be thermophilic *Actinomycete* organisms. Some ventilation systems have also been shown to be sources of amoebae, which thrive in stagnant water, and they or their products may then be inhaled in aerosols.

In Japan, HP occurs during the summer when affected individuals inhale house dust contaminated with *Trichosporon cutaneum*. This summertime HP is the most prevalent type in Japan. The *T. cutaneum* organism has been found only in houses of affected patients and not controls, and a high titer of antibodies was found in patients with the disease.

Animal proteins are another important group of antigens. Avian proteins may be inhaled from the dried excrement of pigeons, doves, ducks, chickens, parakeets, or lovebirds. Between 7% and 15% of individuals caring for the birds become ill after repeated exposure. This disease may also progress to fibrotic lung disease.

Reactive low-molecular-weight volatile chemicals (e.g., isocyanates or phthalic anhydride) that are used in the plastics industry may act as haptens when inhaled or may alter respiratory protein structure, forming new antigens that cause sensitization and subsequent HP. Examples of industrial exposures include polyurethane foam production, paint spraying, and injection molding in foundries.

Various medications (e.g., amiodarone, gold, β-blockers, sulfonamides, nitrofurantoin, chlorambucil, minocycline, and procarbazine) have been associated with pulmonary diseases resembling HP. Methotrexate, tocainide, mexiletine, flecainide, and nonsteroidal anti-inflammatory drugs have also been associated with lung disease. Nitrofurantoin and bleomycin likely cause severe lung damage through a toxic effect mediated by oxygen-derived radicals. Acute nitrofurantoin-hypersensitivity reactions have also been reported.

It is likely that with increased recognition of potential sources of antigens, the number of inhaled organic dusts able to sensitize susceptible individuals will be expanded.

Clinical Features

The clinical features of HP depend on several factors: 1) the nature (particle size, solubility, antigenicity) of the inhaled dust, 2) the intensity and frequency of inhalation exposure, and 3) the type and intensity of the immunologic response of the patient. Another factor that may be important in the induction of disease (as suggested by case histories and demonstrated by experiments) is the concomitant occurrence of pulmonary inflammation, such as a respiratory infection.

Features of the clinical illness are usually similar regardless of the inhaled organic dust, and HP is a syndrome in which there may be a spectrum of clinical signs and symptoms rather than a single, specific pattern (Table 8.2).

Table 8.2 Characteristics of Hypersensitivity Pneumonitis

	Acute	Chronic
Symptoms	Chills, fever, dyspnea, dry cough, malaise 4–6 h after exposure	Progressive dyspnea, cough, malaise, weight loss, anorexia weakness
Examination	Ill, end-inspiratory rales	Dry crackles
Chest radiograph	Normal to interstitial infiltrates	Diffuse interstitial fibrosis
Spirometry	Restriction	Restriction, obstruction, or both
Diffusing capacity	Decreased	Decreased
Bronchoalveolar lavage	Lymphocytic alveolitis	Lymphocytic infiltrate CD8+
Lung biopsy	Interstitial pneumonitis with lymphocytes, histiocytes	Diffuse interstitial fibrosis and noncaseating granulomas
Laboratory	Leukocytosis, elevated erythro-cyte sedimentation rate; serum precipitins present	Normal leukocytes; serum precipitins present
Reversibility	Good	Poor

Acute Form

The clinical features of the acute form of HP are explosive in nature, occurring in temporal relationship to an antigen exposure. The period of sensitization with the offending agent is variable and may take several months or years.

Symptoms are both respiratory and systemic and occur 4 to 6 hours after inhalation exposure once the patient is sensitized. Nonproductive cough, dyspnea, temperature as high as 104°F, chills, myalgia, and malaise are common. The symptoms may persist for 18 to 24 hours; recovery is spontaneous. The attacks recur after each exposure, and the severity of the episode depends on the degree of exposure as well as the sensitivity of the individual. The attacks mimic an acute viral disease, such as influenza, and broad spectrum antibiotic therapy has been administered to these patients for suspected bronchitis or bronchopneumonia. Additional symptoms of anorexia, weight loss, and progressive dyspnea may be prominent with frequent and severe attacks. The symptoms usually resolve within 12 to 18 hours, although they may persist for several days. A common scenario is a patient who improves within a day or two in the hospital while on antibiotics for an atypical pneumonia only to experience symptoms hours to days after rechallenge at home or the workplace.

Chronic Form

In some patients with HP, prolonged exposure may result in irreversible pulmonary damage and progressive respiratory disease, without the acute explosive episodes. Symptoms of cough, malaise, weakness, anorexia, weight loss, and progressive dyspnea on exertion are common and are often the result of prolonged and continuous exposure to small amounts of antigen. Fever is often not present. This form is common in bird breeders who keep birds in the home or in some patients with ventilation pneumonitis who are continuously exposed to a contaminated system.

Physical Examination

Examination of the patient during an acute attack of HP reveals an acutely ill, febrile, dyspneic individual. Bibasilar end-inspiratory rales are prominent and may persist for several hours, days, or weeks after an episode subsides. Between attacks, the examination may be completely normal. In the chronic form, features of interstitial fibrosis are seen with crackling bibasilar rales, nail clubbing, dyspnea, and cyanosis.

Laboratory Features

A leukocytosis as high as 20,000 to 30,000/mm^3 with marked left shift and up to 10% eosinophilia may be present, although eosinophilia is usually absent. All isotypes of immunoglobulin usually are elevated, except IgE. Elevations in erythrocyte sedimentation rate and c-reactive protein have been seen in some cases. In the acute form, arterial blood gases often demonstrate a respiratory alkalosis with hypoxemia. In the chronic form, the hypoxemia is accentuated by exercise.

The immunologic finding characteristic of HP is the demonstration of serum-precipitating antibodies against the specific offending organic dust antigen. Gel diffusion or immunoelectrophoretic techniques can be used to detect antibodies in nearly all ill individuals but also in the serum of as many as 50% of asymptomatic individuals similarly exposed. These tests are rarely negative in HP, but not all antigens for all circumstances are available; thus, individualizing for a given patient's environment may be needed.

Cell-mediated immunity to the offending agent has been demonstrated in patients with HP. Lymphocyte transformation and the production of macrophage migration inhibition factor have been detected in patients with "bird-breeder's disease" but not in their asymptomatic counterparts. The advent of pulmonary lavage has allowed the study of the milieu in which the antigen–antibody cell interaction takes place.

Chest radiograph examination may be within normal limits if the acute attacks are widely spaced. More commonly, in the patient with HP, there are demonstrable fine, sharp modulations and reticulation with general coarsening of bronchovascular markings. During the acute attack, soft, patchy, ill-defined parenchymal densities that tend to coalesce may be seen in the lung fields (Fig. 8.4). End–stage disease may appear on a radiograph as diffuse fibrosis, with parenchymal contraction or even honey-combing. High-resolution CT scans of the chest are no better than conventional radiography in acute HP and can appear similar to desquamative interstitial pneumonia. CT is superior in distinguishing normal from abnormal parenchyma in chronic disease and may show centrilobular nodules; scattered small, round ground-glass opacities; and emphysema–features that are helpful in distinguishing HP from idiopathic pulmonary fibrosis (17). In distinguishing pulmonary sar-

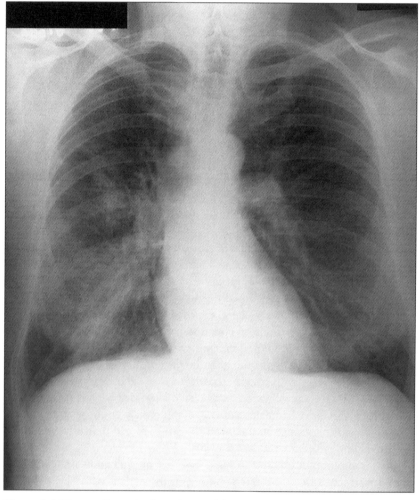

Figure 8.4 Chest radiograph of a patient with hypersensitivity pneumonitis. Bilateral interstitial infiltrates are evident. Note the absence of pleural effusion, hilar adenopathy, and hyperinflation.

coidosis from HP, nodules tend to be bronchocentric in HP rather than following bronchovascular bundles as in pulmonary sarcoidosis. A small series of patients with biopsy-proven infiltrative lung disease have been studied with magnetic resonance imaging. Although generalized, parenchymal opacification (active inflammation) and reticulation (fibrosis) could be identified; localized areas of reticulation and honey-combing are best identified with high-resolution CT.

Pulmonary function abnormalities may be demonstrated during the acute episode of HP. The most common response occurs 4 to 6 hours after exposure and is a decrease in FVC and FEV_1, with little alteration of their ratio. There is little change in expiratory flow rates. A decrease in compliance, indicating an increased lung stiffness, and decreased diffusion capacity also occur. These abnormalities resolve as the attack subsides. With sufficient parenchymal damage, however, the pulmonary function abnormalities in volume and flow may be found during asymptomatic phases, and hypoxia and hypercapnia may also be detected. In chronic HP, a predominately restrictive ventilatory impairment with a decrease in diffusing capacity is seen.

A second type of response, which has been observed in patients with pigeon-protein sensitivity (and rarely with *Actinomycete* sensitivity), occurs in two stages. There is an immediate asthmatic response with a decrease in FVC, FEV_1, and expiratory flow rates. This response is then followed by a late reaction.

It is important to recognize differences between the late phase of the dual asthmatic response as seen in atopic individuals and the late phase of the respiratory response of HP. In asthma, the late phase is primarily obstructive with a decrease in FEV_1, FEV_1:FVC ratio and flow, but not FVC. The diffusing capacity does not change. In the late phase of HP, a decrease in FVC and FEV_1 occurs, with little change in the FEV_1:FVC ratio. With a severe, restrictive defect, the expiratory flow rates may also decrease. The diffusing capacity also decreases and, if the reaction is severe, hypoxemia may be observed.

Bronchoalveolar Lavage

Lung lavage of normal individuals reveals low total numbers of cells with predominately alveolar macrophages and lymphocytes. The vast majority of the lymphocytes are T cells, with a tendency toward CD8+ suppresser cells compared with CD4+ helper cells. Cigarette smoking can cause an alveolitis characterized by a three- to five-fold increase in numbers and activation of macrophages, along with a small increase in neutrophils.

Lung lavage of pigeon breeders contains relatively high titers of specific IgG and IgA antibodies, and titers of IgA may be higher in symptomatic than in healthy breeders.

The cellular components of lung fluids in HP have marked increases in lymphocytes, predominately T cells of the CD8+ or suppresser type. Activated lung macrophages and enhanced cell function are also seen, and increases in mast cells and natural killer cells are evident. T-cell elevations have also been seen in both symptomatic and asymptomatic individuals, which suggests that a subclinical form of the disease may also result from exposure to organic dust antigens. Lung lymphocytes stimulated with specific antigen demonstrate increased blastogenic activity in ill but not in well individuals. In the presence of specific antigen, this pulmonary lymphocyte blastogenesis correlates better with disease activity than does peripheral cellular or humoral studies.

Histopathology

Although the offending antigen may be quite different, most varieties of HP are characterized by similar histologic changes. These changes largely depend on the intensity of antigen exposure and the stage of the disease during which the biopsy is performed. In acute HP, the reaction is confined to alveolar and interstitial inflammation, with predominance of lymphocytes, activated macrophages, plasma cells, and neutrophils. In HP, macrophages with foamy cytoplasm are a frequent pathologic feature that suggests activation.

In the chronic stage, changes include lymphocytic alveolitis, intra-alveolar foamy macrophages, increases in mast cells and plasma cells, interstitial inflammation, noncaseating granulomas, intra-alveolar buds, and interstitial fibrosis (Fig. 8.5). Most biopsies revealed granulomas that differ from those found in sarcoidosis by appearing smaller, more loosely arranged, poorly limited with a higher predominance of lymphocytes, and more frequently located in alveolar tissue than in the vicinity of bronchioles and vessels. The severity of fibrosis is variable and associated with relatively little epithelial cell necrosis or connective tissue destruction, which suggests a reparative stage of an exudative process. Even in the late stages of HP, characteristic features seen in early stages are present. This may distinguish HP from idiopathic pulmonary fibrosis.

Immunopathogenesis

Hypersensitivity pneumonitis is accepted as an immunologic disorder; the exact mechanisms involved in the pathogenesis have not been clarified, and there may be multiple immunologic and even non-immunologic influences on the disease, depending on the stage.

Hypersensitivity pneumonitis is characterized by lung interstitium and epithelial surface inflammation, and the sequence of events of the inflammatory

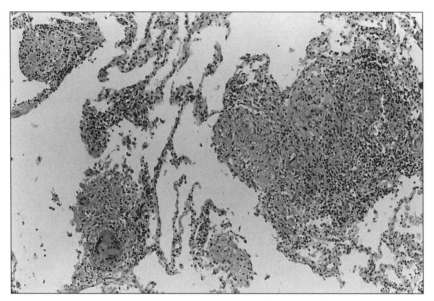

Figure 8.5 Lung biopsy of a patient with hypersensitivity pneumonitis that demonstrates diffuse lymphocytic infiltrate with noncaseating granulomata.

process is likely multifaceted. The initial presentation follows repeated antigen exposure at the terminal bronchioles and alveolar level. Presumably, antigen-processing cells engulf and process the antigen and release cytokines. Such processing may be lengthy, with engulfed particulate dusts. The cytokines are likely responsible for the ensuing cellular infiltration. A variety of such inflammatory molecules have been detected in the bronchoalveolar lavage (BAL) of patients (15). CD8+ lymphocytes and activation of other T cells have also been detected. In the acute phase of HP, there is a marked increase in polymorphonuclear leukocytes (probably cytokine mediated) found within the alveoli.

The acute inflammatory response then resolves with a fall in polymorphonuclear cells, but the quantity of total cells recovered in the BAL continues to be elevated, with a predominance of lymphocytes, which may then continue throughout the disease process. The alveolar macrophage and lymphocytes are thus probably the primary effector cells. Activated macrophages also release chemoattractants and cytokines that enhance lymphocyte migration. Other cytokines, such as IL-1 and IL-2, may be important in inducing the lymphocytic alveolitis. The mechanism of the initiation and maintenance of the granulomatous response of HP likely is due to the dynamic interaction between the inciting agent, the release of inflammatory mediators, attraction of leukocytes, and the resident structural cells.

Host factors play a role in the pathogenesis of the disease, because the majority of individuals exposed to organic dusts remain asymptomatic. Comparing the two exposed populations has provided some information regarding susceptibility. Significantly higher levels of IgE, IgM, and IgA in epithelial lining fluid as well as specific antibody levels against antigen have been shown in ill individuals. Neither atopy nor HLA haplotypes correlate with susceptibility to HP. Tobacco smoking appears to have a negative influence on total and functional lung immunoglobulin that is not permanent; tobacco smoking may also interfere with alveolar macrophage function and processing of antigen.

Diagnosis

The diagnosis of HP should be considered in patients with intermittent pulmonary and systemic symptoms or with progressive, unexplained pulmonary symptoms and evidence for interstitial lung disease. A carefully obtained history detailing possible temporal relationships between symptoms and an occupation, hobby, or use of forced-air equipment may provide clues. No single clinical or diagnostic laboratory test is available, and in the final analysis a combination of clinical findings, radiographic abnormalities, pulmonary function, and immunologic testing supports the diagnosis. Inhalational challenge and lung biopsy may be necessary in some cases to confirm the disease. Laboratory findings may be helpful, particularly in the acute stages during which findings may include elevated erythrocyte sedimentation rate, positive c-reactive protein, increased leukocyte count, and arterial hypoxemia.

Immunologic studies of the patient's sera, using available antigens of thermophilic *Actinomycetes* organisms, *Aspergillus* species, or avian proteins in a gel-diffusion system, may confirm exposure but not necessarily disease. False-negative HP reports may stem from improper quality controls, insensitive techniques, or use of the wrong antigen or under-concentrated sera. An accurate and reliable reference laboratory may avoid the need for expensive or invasive procedures. Additional antigen preparations that have been made from dusts or fungi cultured from the furnace humidifier or the place of employment may be needed to detect an immunologic reaction. Antigen skin testing has little practical role, because both false-positive and -negative reactions can occur.

Although results of pulmonary function tests and chest radiograph examination may vary, depending on whether the evaluation is during an acute episode or in the chronic stage of the disease; they may be normal if the patient is studied in an asymptomatic period. When a specific environment is suspected as the cause of the patient's symptoms, it may be necessary to perform pulmonary function tests before and several hours after exposure. If significant changes occur in vital capacity, diffusing capacity, or even flow rates, the environment should be suspected and further investigated with cultures and immunologic studies.

Potential indications for a high-resolution chest CT include 1) normal or nonspecific findings on a chest radiograph, 2) further evaluation of lung parenchyma in patients whose chest films are inconsistent with the clinical history or symptomatology, 3) as a guide to an optimal lung biopsy site, and 4) to detect suspected complications when clinical or lung functions deteriorate despite treatment.

Inhalation challenge using suspected antigenic materials should be done in a hospital laboratory because of the potential of severe reactions. The amount of antigen used for insufflation challenge is arbitrary, because there is no way to judge the sensitivity or possible reactivity of each patient other than by history. Patients are given 2 mL of a 1:10 weight-to-volume extract of fungal or *Actinomycete* culture filtrate over 15 minutes by means of an oxygen-powered nebulizer; patients should be examined hourly with pulmonary function tests, leukocyte counts, and temperature measurements. In this manner, the acute attack can be reproduced, and corticosteroids may be used to abort a severe episode. Episodes of pneumonitis provoked in the laboratory usually resolve in a few hours, unlike the spontaneous episode that may last many days.

Bronchoscopy with alveolar lavage may help distinguish HP from sarcoid lung by evaluating T-helper-cell subsets CD4+ and CD8+. A predominance of CD8+ suppresser cells suggests HP.

Lung biopsy should be carried out only if the other diagnostic efforts do not establish the diagnosis. Because the histopathologic features of HP are not entirely specific, they must be considered in light of the entire case.

Differential Diagnosis

Several other syndromes should be considered when evaluating patients for HP. The possibilities differ depending on the environment of the particular individual. Building-related illnesses can induce symptoms by several mechanisms, including immunologic, infectious, toxic, or irritant (16). Febrile illnesses occurring after inhalation of organic dusts have been recognized for years, particularly by agricultural workers, and can be difficult to differentiate from HP. Building-associated illness includes "sick-building" syndrome, which is rather vague and subjective, and "building-related" illnesses, which are relatively well-characterized human illnesses. The "sick-building" syndrome appears to result from increased demand for energy conservation in heated and air-conditioned office buildings. To reduce energy costs, intermixing of fresh and recirculated air is reduced to a minimum. The concentration of a variety of multiple contaminants (usually volatile organic chemicals and microbes, which are ordinarily reduced by adequate ventilation interchange) is increased. Up to 90% of the inhabitants of the building develop irritative ocular and respiratory symptoms. Other vague and predominately subjective complaints include neurobehavioral symptoms, such as memory loss, headache, depression, dizziness, and respiratory complaints (e.g., chest tightness, coughing, and shortness of breath). Anxiety levels increase in the workers, but other clinical findings are uncommon. Recognition and correction of the extreme energy-conservation measures usually resolves the situation.

The organic dust toxic syndrome (ODTS) refers to the group of noninfectious febrile illnesses described by various terms, including pulmonary mycotoxicosis, "silo-unloader's" disease, grain fever, mill fever, humidifier fever, and "animal-house" fever (17). It occurs in workers after exposure to agricultural dusts and toxins generated from organic materials contaminated with multiple bacterial and fungal species. The ODTS is 30 to 50 times more common in farmers than HP. It occurs more commonly in the summer months and among individuals younger than those with HP.

Humidifier fever occurs where recirculated water is sprayed into the air for humidification or cooling or for cleaning manufacturing equipment. The water becomes contaminated with gram-negative organisms that produce endotoxins. Affected workers develop fever, malaise, and mild cough, with chest tightness 4 to 8 hours after exposure. Chest radiographs are normal and pulmonary function tests are either normal or show mild airway obstruction without impairment of gas transfer. The symptoms clear completely in a few hours. Serologic tests may be positive for microbial antigens from the environment, but inhalation challenges with these antigens do not consistently reproduce symptoms. Inhalation of endotoxins, however, does provoke effects in approximately half of previously unexposed volunteers (18).

Grain dust and dust in swine confinement and poultry-raising buildings as well as in laboratory animal quarters can cause similar symptoms (e.g., grain fever, toxic organic dust syndromes). The respiratory symptoms are not due solely to endotoxins but are related to ammonia and hydrogen sulfide gases generated by animal excrement. Lung biopsies or bronchoalveolar lavage data have not been reported in inhaled endotoxins. In patients with ODTS, BAL fluid has shown increased numbers of total cells, polymorphonuclear cells, and spore and fungal elements. A predominately CD8+ lymphocytic alveolitis can be seen after the first week. Inflammation of the airways may predominate.

Chronic exposure to cotton dust causes the chronic obstructive lung disease byssinosis. Cotton dust is a complex mixture of biologic agents, including a histamine-releasing factor, tannins, and endotoxins. Endotoxins in cotton dust likely contributes to the acute symptoms of byssinosis or "Monday-morning" fever.

Dense clouds of mold spores, which farmers may inhale while forking off the top layer of a silo or cleaning a dry silo in preparation for the new crop, can cause pulmonary mycotoxicosis—a bilateral, widespread, acute pneumonitis. Cultures of lung biopsies taken during this acute pneumonitis grow large numbers of a variety of fungi, but the acute disease is quite different from farmer's lung. The typical serology is absent and lung biopsy lacks granulomata. Response is related to clearing the organisms and the use of appropriate pharmacotherapeutic agents.

In the differential diagnosis of chronic HP, one should consider the conditions that may cause interstitial lung disease with resultant progressive pulmonary and systemic symptoms. Distinguishing characteristics that suggest sarcoidosis include hilar adenopathy; elevated serum angiotensin-converting–enzyme level; subtle differences in histopathology; CD4+ T-cell alveolitis; and positive Gallium scan, with involvement of parotid gland, lymph nodes, and extrathoracic tissues. Primary pulmonary histiocytosis in contrast to HP is characterized by 10% spontaneous pneumothorax, wheezing, hemoptysis, and Langerhans' cells in BAL fluid and on open lung biopsy. Gallium scans are usually negative, and in most large series, almost all patients with histiocytosis were current or former smokers. Idiopathic pulmonary fibrosis is differentiated from HP by clubbing on physical examination and, frequently, an aggressive fatal outcome within 6 years after onset. However, by means of environmental and immunologic studies—along with close observation of the patient during periods of exposure and avoidance—the appropriate diagnosis can be made.

Treatment

As in other allergic respiratory diseases, treatment of HP includes avoidance of the offending antigen. Once the antigen is identified, a variety of precautions may be attempted. The use of air-filtering systems, masks, or alterations in forced-air heating or cooling systems may be of benefit. In some cases, a change in hobbies or occupations may be necessary. In general, in acute disease, the majority of individuals can expect complete resolution of symptoms and a return to normal pulmonary function days to weeks after the exposure has stopped and if irreversible pulmonary damage has not occurred.

Environmental changes (e.g., improved ventilation in pigeon coops, wearing protective respirators, changing farming techniques, and withdrawal of suspected drugs) may be important therapeutic measures.

In the event a drug is the suspected agent inducing HP, withdrawal of such drug along with suppression of any pulmonary inflammatory reaction is indicated.

Pharmacologic measures should be used if the offending antigen cannot be avoided or if the disease appears to be progressing even with avoidance. Antihistamines are generally not effective. Albuterol has shown to be helpful in challenge studies in which there is an acute fall in FEV_1, and cromolyn sodium has been reported to prevent symptoms in the laboratory. There is no evidence that these drugs can prevent acute or chronic disease when used during times of natural exposure. Oral corticosteroids remain the mainstay of therapy in patients with HP, and the clinical and laboratory responses to these drugs are often dramatic. The duration of therapy should be judged on the basis of clinical and laboratory improvement; however, avoidance is still of utmost importance, and one should not rely on corticosteroid therapy to suppress symptoms. Immunotherapy with the offending antigens is not advisable because of potential adverse effects from injected microbial toxins or the development of immune-complex vasculitis.

Reversal of the disease process depends on how quickly the diagnosis is made so that avoidance, drug therapy, or both may be instituted. The clinical and laboratory abnormalities generally revert to normal after a variable period of therapy, unless pulmonary damage has become irreversible; therefore, early detection of clinical illness and identification and subsequent avoidance of the offending environmental antigen are most important.

REFERENCES

1. **Rosenberg MR, Patterson R, Mintzer R, et al.** Clinical and immunologic criteria for the diagnosis of allergic bronchopulmonary aspergillosis. Ann Intern Med. 1977;86: 405-14.

2. **Greenberger PA, Patterson R.** Diagnosis and management of allergic bronchopulmonary aspergillosis. Ann Allergy. 1986;56:444-53.

3. **Patterson R, Greenberger PA, Halwig JM, et al.** Allergic bronchopulmonary aspergillosis: natural history and classification of early disease by serologic and roentgenographic studies. Arch Intern Med. 1986;146:916-8.

4. **Wang JLF, Patterson R, Rosenberg M, et al.** Serum IgE and IgG antibody activity against *Aspergillus fumigatus* as a diagnostic aid in allergic bronchopulmonary aspergillosis. Am Rev Resp Dis. 1978;117:917-27.

5. **Mintzer RA, Rogers CF, Kruglik GD.** The spectrum of radiologic findings in ABPA. Radiology. 1978;127:301-7.

6. **Neeld DA, Goodman LR, Gurney JW, et al.** Computerized tomography in the evaluation of ABPA. Am Rev Resp Dis. 1990;142:1200-5.

7. **Safirstein BH, D'Souza MF, Simon G, et al.** Five-year follow-up of allergic bronchopulmonary aspergillosis. Am Rev Resp Dis. 1973;108:450-9.

8. **Patterson R, Greenberger PA, Radin RC, Roberts M.** Allergic bronchopulmonary aspergillosis: staging as an aid to management. Ann Int Med. 1982;96:286-91.

9. **Laufer P, Fink JN, Bruns WT, et al.** Allergic bronchopulmonary aspergillosis in cystic fibrosis. J Allergy Clin Immunol. 1984;73:44-8.

10. **Knutsen AP, Mueller KR, Levine AD, et al.** *Asp fI* CD4+TH2-like T-cell lines in allergic bronchopulmonary aspergillosis. J Allergy Clin Immunol. 1994;94:215-21.

11. **Knutsen AP, Mueller KR, Hutcheson PS, Slavin RG.** T-and B-cell dysregulation of

IgE synthesis in cystic fibrosis patients with allergic bronchopulmonary aspergillosis. Clin Immunol Immunopathol. 1990;55:128–38.

12. **Rickett AJ, Greenberger PA, Patterson R.** Serum IgE as an important aid in management of allergic bronchopulmonary aspergillosis. J Allergy Clin Immunol. 1984; 74:68–71.

13. **Lopez M, Salvaggio JE.** Epidemiology of hypersensitivity pneumonitis/allergic alveolitis. Monogr Allergy. 1987;21:70–86.

14. **Banaszak EF, Thiede WH, Fink JN.** Hypersensitivity pneumonitis due to contamination of an air conditioner. N Engl J Med. 1970;283:271–6.

15. **Walker C, Bauer W, Braun RK, et al.** Activated T cells and cytokines in bronchoalveolar lavages from patients with various lung diseases associated with eosinophilia. Am J Resp Crit Care Med. 1994;150:1038–48.

16. **Seltzer JM.** Building-related illnesses. J Allergy Clin Immunol. 1994;94:351–62.

17. **Parker JE, Petsonk LE, Weber SL.** Hypersensitivity pneumonitis and organic dust toxic syndrome. Immunol Allergy Clin North Am. 1992;12:279–90.

18. **Rylander R, Bake B, Fischer JJ, Helander IM.** Pulmonary function and symptoms after inhalation of endotoxin. Am Rev Respir Dis. 1989;140:981–6.

SUGGESTING READINGS

Allergic Bronchopulmonary Aspergillosis

Graves TS, Fink JN, Patterson R, et al. A familial occurrence of allergic bronchopulmonary aspergillosis. Ann Int Med. 1978;91:378–82.

Katzenstein AL, Trebow A, Friedman P. Bronchocentric granulomatosis, mucoid impaction, and hypersensitivity reactions to fungi. Am Rev Resp Dis. 1975;111:497–537.

Kurup VP, Kumar A. Immunodiagnosis of aspergillosis. Clin Microbiol Rev. 1991;4: 439–56.

Kurup VP, Greenberger PA, Fink JN. Antibody response to low-molecular-weight antigens of *Aspergillus fumigatus* in allergic bronchopulmonary aspergillosis. J Clin Microbiol. 1989;27:1312–6.

Moser M, Crameri R, Brust E, et al. Diagnostic value of recombinant *Aspergillus fumigatus* allergen I/a for skin testing and serology. J Allergy Clin Immunol. 1994;93:1–11.

Patterson R, Greenberger PA, Lee TM, et al. Prolonged evaluation of patients with corticosteroid-dependent asthma stage of allergic bronchopulmonary aspergillosis. J Allergy Clin Immunol. 1987;80:663–8.

Hypersensitivity Pneumonitis

Fink JN. Hypersensitivity pneumonitis. Clin Chest Med. 1992;13:303–9.

Kaltreider HB. Hypersensitivity pneumonitis. West J Med. 1993;159:570–8.

Salvaggio JE. Inhaled particles and respiratory disease. J Allergy Clin Immunol. 1994;94: 304–9.

Salvaggio JE, Millhollon BW. Allergic alveolitis: new insights into old mysteries. Resp Med. 1993;87:495–501.

Chapter 9

Immunodeficiencies

Robert P. Nelson, Jr., MD

Immunodeficiency states in adults are characterized clinically by recurrent infections, persistent infections, and infections with organisms of low virulence. Primary immunodeficiency disorders result from a failure of development and maturation of components of the immune system. Secondary immunodeficiencies occur when the body's defenses are limited by altered physiologic states attributable to illness, age, malnutrition, or adverse effects of medical therapies. Primary immunodeficiencies result from defects that are generally hereditary and congenital and are usually diagnosed during infancy or childhood (1). Internists may encounter patients with primary immunodeficiency diseases in at least three situations. First, disorders such as common variable immunodeficiency present most commonly during adulthood; second, mild phenotypic variants of disorders that present initially in childhood may not be noted until adulthood; and, third, with improvements in treatment, children with a variety of immunodeficiencies now survive to adulthood (Box 9.1) (2). The increased recognition of primary immunodeficiency diseases in adults and the broad array of disease states that result in susceptibility to recurrent infections make immunodeficiency syndromes some of the most common conditions that the internist must understand, recognize, and manage.

Box 9.1 Primary Immunodeficiencies in Adults

Initial clinical presentation in adult life
  IgA deficiency
  Common variable immunodeficiency
  IgG subclass deficiency
  Complement deficiencies
  Antibody deficiency with normal immunoglobulins
Delayed presentation of a disorder typical of childhood
  Adenosine deaminase deficiency
  Wiskott–Aldrich syndrome
  X-linked agammaglobulinemia
  Chronic granulomatous disease
  Purine nucleoside phosphorylase deficiency
Disorders with childhood onset and survival into adulthood
  Severe combined immunodeficiency disease
  Chronic granulomatous disease
  X-linked agammaglobulinemia
  Ommen syndrome
  X-linked lymphoproliferative disease
  Wiskott–Aldrich syndrome
  Immunoglobulin deficiency with increased IgM

Normal immunologic function relies primarily on the successful interaction of four components: B lymphocytes, T lymphocytes, phagocytic cells, and complement components. Defective development of B lymphocytes results in abnormalities in humoral immunity and increased susceptibility to pyogenic infections of high-grade encapsulated bacterial pathogens. Deficient T-cell function is associated classically with increased susceptibility to infection from opportunistic pathogens. Phagocytic disorders include abnormalities in neutrophil number and function and are associated with increased frequency and severity of bacterial and fungal infections. Rare deficiencies related to the absence of specific complement components result in increased susceptibility to infections and autoimmune disease. Systemic illness may affect one or more of these components and includes diabetes, malignancy, and infectious diseases (e.g., HIV infection; malnutrition; and states induced by chemotherapy, immunosuppressive therapy, radiation, and following solid-organ and bone marrow transplantation). This chapter summarizes the primary and secondary immunodeficiencies, concentrating on those illnesses that affect adults.

Box 9.2 Primary Antibody Deficiencies

IgA deficiency
Common variable immunodeficiency (hyper-IgM)
X-linked agammaglobulinemia
Immunoglobulin deficiency with increased IgM
Selective deficiency of IgG subclasses
Antibody deficiency with normal immunoglobulin

Primary Immunodeficiency Diseases

Antibody Deficiencies

Primary antibody-deficiency diseases are a group of congenital or acquired conditions in which recurrent bacterial and viral infections occur as a consequence of impaired antibody production (Box 9.2).

IgA Deficiency
Isolated IgA deficiency occurs with a frequency of 1 in 400 persons and is more prevalent in whites than in blacks and in Asians.

Clinical Manifestations: A large number of reports have linked selective IgA deficiency with recurrent infections, gastrointestinal disease, allergic diathesis, and autoimmune conditions; however, the prevalence of isolated IgA deficiency is no different in hospital-based compared with community-based surveys of healthy individuals. Most persons with IgA deficiency are clinically normal. Upper respiratory infections are the primary clinical manifestation in those that experience symptoms. Patients with severe or lower respiratory infection generally have a broader-based deficiency, such as an IgG2 or IgG4 subclass deficiency or common variable immunodeficiency (3).

Case 9.1

A 19-year-old white man presented with a history of recurrent upper respiratory infections and sinusitis over the past 2 to 3 years. During the course of 1 year, he was hospitalized with two episodes of pneumonia, which resolved with appropriate intravenous antibacterial therapy directed toward community-acquired organisms. Past medical history was significant for idiopathic thrombocytopenic purpura at 13 years of age. A maternal aunt had been diagnosed with systemic lupus erythematosus. Review of systems was significant for intermittent diarrhea. *Continued*

Case 9.1 (continued)

The patient was in the 25th percentile for height, 10th for weight. His blood pressure, pulse rate, body temperature, and respiratory rate were all normal for his age. He had dark rings under the eyes (allergic shiners), a green-yellow nasal discharge, bilateral nasal mucosal edema, and postnasal drip visible in the posterior pharynx. Bilateral fine crackles in the bases were present on forced expiration. Results from cardiac, rectal, neurologic, and skin examinations were normal. Abdominal examination revealed palpable spleen tip. Hemoccult results were negative. The patient had bilateral cervical and axillary adenopathy. His extremities exhibited no cyanosis or clubbing.

Complete blood count revealed white blood count at 13,600 (75% polymorphonuclear leukocytes, 22% lymphocytes, 3% monocytes), hemoglobin 12.5 g/dL, hematocrit 35.4, and platelets 290,000/mm³. Waters–Caldwell view of the maxillary sinus revealed bilateral opacification of the maxillary and ethmoid sinuses. The chest radiograph showed no abnormalities. An immunologic evaluation was warranted because of the patient's high frequency of sinus infections and pneumonia. Serum IgG levels were 150 mg/dL (528–2190 mg/dL), IgA levels were less than 7 mg/dL (44–441 mg/dL), and IgM levels were 15 mg/dL (48–226 mg/dL). Tetanus, diphtheria, and pneumococcal titers were not protective, despite previous immunizations. Serum protein electrophoresis showed hypogammaglobulin without evidence for monoclonal gammopathy. CD3+ and T-lymphocyte percentage was 70% (55%–72%), CD4+ was 47% (35%–55%), and CD8+ was 21% (18%–32%).

This patient is a young adult with recurrent upper respiratory infection and sinusitis. Under these circumstances, recurrent infections and sinusitis are most often related to viral upper respiratory infections. Also, allergic diatheses may result in increased susceptibility to infection. Forms of rhinitis (e.g., vasomotor rhinitis, rhinitis medicamentosa, and nonallergic rhinitis with eosinophils) are considerations in people who have upper respiratory infections and sinusitis. When the history includes hospitalizations for two episodes of pneumonia, an immunodeficiency should be considered. One of the most common immunodeficiency diseases associated with recurrent infections of the sinuses is HIV. Other primary antibody deficiencies to consider under these circumstances include IgA deficiency, common variable immunodeficiency, X-linked agammaglobulinemia (in an adult), and antibody deficiency with near normal immunoglobulins. Past medical history is significant for an episode of idiopathic thrombocytopenic purpura and autoimmune phenomena, which does occur with increased frequency in patients with antibody deficiency. In this case, the physical examination is also remarkable for a palpable spleen. Palpable lymph nodes militate against X-linked agammaglobulinemia. The most likely diagnostic entities are HIV, common variable immunodeficiency disease, and IgA deficiency.

The patient demonstrates no ability to make antibodies to Pneumococcus. The preferred treatment in this case of CVID would be intravenous gammaglobulin therapy.

Diagnosis: Diagnosis is established by a serum IgA level less than 5 mg/dL, with normal IgG and IgM levels and normal antibody responses to immunizations of bacterial antigens, such as diphtheria, tetanus, and Pneumococcus.

Treatment: IgA-deficient patients may have IgG or IgE antibodies directed against IgA, which may result in transfusion reactions. A Medic-Alert bracelet should be worn, and washed, packed erythrocytes should be used if transfusion is necessary. Intravenous gammaglobulin is contraindicated for patients with isolated IgA deficiency, because anti-IgA antibodies are capable of producing anaphylactic or anaphylactoid reactions.

Common Variable Immunodeficiency

Common variable immunodeficiency (CVID) is a multisystem disorder of unknown etiology that is characterized by antibody deficiency, autoimmune manifestations, and an increased risk of malignancies. CVID is the most common clinically significant primary immunodeficiency that often presents initially in adult life (4). It occurs with a frequency of 1 in 75,000 population, with equal distribution between men and women. It occurs at any age between infancy and old age, with peak incidences between 6 and 10 years of age and also between 26 and 30 years of age. The cause of CVID appears to be related to an intrinsic abnormality in the terminal differentiation of B cells to antibody-secreting plasma cells. Approximately one half of CVID patients have decreased T-cell proliferative responses to antigens.

Clinical Manifestations: Patients develop recurrent pyogenic infections of the upper and lower respiratory tract. These are commonly caused by encapsulated bacteria (e.g., *Haemophilus influenzae*, *Streptococcus pneumoniae*, *Staphylococcus aureus*, *Pseudomonas aeruginosa*), unencapsulated *H. influenzae*, and *Mycoplasma*. Chronic sinusitis is often the initial manifestation; chronic otitis media, bronchitis, and pneumonia also occur. Blood-borne infections are seen with increased frequency, including meningitis, sepsis, septic arthritis, and osteomyelitis. Pulmonary complications include chronic progressive bronchiectasis, interstitial pneumonia, pulmonary insufficiency, and cor pulmonale. In vitro lymphoid proliferation results in lymphoid hyperplasia, with infiltration of organs or tissues. Infection from opportunistic organisms in patients with CVID is less common but does occur with increased frequency compared with healthy individuals. These organisms include *Pneumocystis carinii*, herpes zoster, and a variety of fungi. Susceptibility to tuberculosis is increased.

Chronic diarrhea occurs in up to 50% of patients with CVID and may be secondary to nodular lymphoid hyperplasia, bacterial overgrowth, or infections with *Giardia lamblia*, *Campylobacter jejuni*, rotavirus, *Salmonella*, or *Shigella*. A sprue-like syndrome occurs in some patients who experience malabsorption and steatorrhea. Ulcerative colitis, Crohn's disease, and chronic active hepatitis occur with increased frequency. Autoimmune manifestations develop in one third of patients and include hemolytic anemia, sicca syndrome, systemic lupus erythematosus, autoimmune thyroiditis, vitiligo, primary biliary cirrhosis, thrombocytopenia, pernicious anemia, and arthritis. Inflammatory or autoimmune disorders are the initial clinical presentations of some patients with CVID, preceding the onset of infections by years. Lymphocytic hyperplasia results in splenomegaly in most patients and lymphoid interstitial pneumonia in some. Noncaseating granulomatous infiltration (similar to sarcoidosis) occurs in the lung, liver, spleen, and conjunctivae and may result in respiratory insufficiency, hepatosplenomegaly, and iridocyclitis. There is a 6% to 16% incidence of malignancy—predominantly non-Hodgkin's lymphoma and gastrointestinal malignancies.

Diagnosis: The diagnosis of CVID is based on the detection of low immunoglobulin levels and production. Serum IgG levels are below 500 mg/dL, and IgA and IgM levels are usually below normal. IgG subclass levels are variably decreased. All patients are deficient in antibody production to bacterial antigens, which is demonstrated by a failure to respond to immunization to protein (diphtheria, tetanus) and carbohydrate (pneumococcal capsular polysaccharide) antigens. Random antibody titers to diphtheria, tetanus, and *Streptococcus pneumoniae* are generally low, and titers obtained 4 weeks following immunization do not reach protective levels. Most patients have normal B-cell numbers, and T-lymphocyte subpopulations are normal or may demonstrate increased CD8+ lymphocyte numbers.

Common variable immunodeficiency must be distinguished from hypogammaglobulinemia due to protein loss, which is caused by enteropathy or nephropathy when malabsorption and weight loss are present; to make a proper diagnosis, one will have to await successful treatment of these conditions. The differential diagnosis includes hypogammaglobulinemia associated with chronic lymphocytic leukemia, thymoma (Good's syndrome), and other lymphoreticular malignancies; hypogammaglobulinemia secondary to drugs, such as phenytoin or cyclophosphamide; and X-linked agammaglobulinemia that presents relatively late in life. First-degree relatives may have IgA deficiency or autoimmune illness, which suggests a genetic basis for the immunologic dysregulation.

Treatment: Immunoglobulin replacement therapy is the treatment of choice for patients with CVID. The immediate objective of IgG replacement therapy is to decrease the frequency and severity of infections and to improve the quality of life, with the ultimate long-term goal of preventing late complications, such as bronchiectasis, progressive pulmonary insufficiency, and chronic sinusitis. Trough IgG levels obtained before an infusion should be maintained above 500 to 600 mg/dL. Unfortunately, some patients with CVID continue to experience recurrent respiratory infections, which progress to bronchiectasis and pulmonary insufficiency despite intravenous immunoglobulin (IVIG) treatment begun before the development of pulmonary symptoms. Early and aggressive antimicrobial therapy for the treatment of infection is indicated. Prophylactic antibiotic therapy reduces the frequency of infection during a 3- to 6-month period within the first phase of immunoglobulin replacement therapy.

An occasional patient with CVID, borderline immunoglobulin levels, and mild clinical phenotype may be managed with prophylactic antibiotics. These patients will require IVIG should infections or chronic diarrhea ensue; pulmonary function should be monitored yearly. Chronic sinusitis is a frequent problem in patients with CVID. Symptoms include nasal congestion, mucopurulent discharge, postnasal drip, cough that is often worse at night, and malodorous breath, with or without fever. Patients should have antibiotics at home and should begin treatment when signs of a mucopurulent discharge ensue. Amoxicillin, amoxicillin clavulanic acid, trimethoprim–sulfamethoxazole, or a second-generation cephalosporin (e.g., cefuroxime or loracarbef) is given for 2 to 4 weeks to eradicate the common pathogens, including *H. influenzae, Streptococcus pneumoniae*, and *Branhamella catarrhalis*. Clindamycin or ciprofloxacin is an alternative for treatment failures. Otolaryngologic evaluation with endoscopic sinus aspiration is recommended to define the pathogen and its antimicrobial sensitivities for patients who do not improve. Intravenous antibiotic therapy with ticarcillin–clavulinic acid, cefuroxime, ceftazidime, or clindamycin will help some patients who do not get better with oral therapy. Endoscopic sinus surgery may be required to remove chronic inflammatory sinus tissue and relieve osteomeatal obstruction as an adjunct to medical therapy. The treatment of chronic draining otitis media requires antibiotic therapy directed at the specific organism; middle-ear culture is recommended. In addition to the organisms above, *Staphylococcus aureus* and *Pseudomonas aeruginosa* are found.

Recurrent bronchitis and pneumonia often respond to antimicrobial therapy directed at community-acquired organisms. Patients with bronchiectasis should be treated when exacerbations are heralded by change in sputum character. Infection with *P. aeruginosa* is treated with oral quinolones, intravenous aminoglycoside, or third-generation cephalosporin therapy. Recalcitrant exacerbations secondary to localized bronchiectasis may require surgical resection. Pulmonary physiotherapy may be a useful adjunct to medical therapy.

Treatment of diarrhea requires the clinician to review the diagnostic possibilities, including infectious diarrhea, bacterial overgrowth, malabsorption secondary to the sprue-like condition, gluten sensitivity, and antibiotic-induced diarrhea (e.g., *Clostridium difficille*). Infection with *G. lamblia* is a common problem and usually responds to metronidazole. Small bowel biopsy is sometimes necessary to establish a diagnosis.

Autoimmune conditions are managed similarly to those in patients without CVID. Surveillance for the occurrence of lymphoma or gastrointestinal carcinomas should include a complete history and physical examination every 6 months and complete blood count, chemistry panel, and hemoccult stool examination yearly or when dictated by clinical status. Chest radiograph is indicated for persistent pulmonary symptoms. Patients with CVID should have the benefit of consultation and follow-up with a subspecialist experienced in the care of these patients. Patients who do not develop malignancy, progressive pulmonary disease, or chronic hepatitis experience good health for extended periods. Accurate figures of life expectancy in the current age of high-dose intravenous replacement therapy are not yet available.

X-Linked Agammaglobulinemia: X-linked agammaglobulinemia (XLA), or Bruton's gammaglobulinemia, is characterized by failure of B-cell maturation and results in profound deficiencies of antibody production. Affected male patients usually present in childhood after the first 6 to 9 months of age, but some are diagnosed as adults. XLA results from mutations in Bruton's tyrosine kinase (BTK), which is expressed in B cells and neutrophils (5). This defect results in maturation arrest at the pre–B-cell stage, resulting in low B-cell numbers and hypogammaglobulinemia. Patients experience recurrent infections of encapsulated organisms similar to those found in CVID. Nontypable *H. influenzae*, a variety of gram-negative bacilli, and *Mycoplasma* are important to those XLA patients who develop chronic lung disease. Bacterial meningitis, sepsis, arthritis, and osteomyelitis occur less often in XLA patients but with a higher frequency than in the normal population. Chronic enteroviral (usually echovirus) meningoencephalitis is a clinical problem that is unique to patients with XLA and may occur despite immunoglobulin therapy.

Diagnosis: When present, a positive family history of recurrent infections in adult male patients or of fatal boyhood infections suggests immunodeficiency. The diagnosis is established by measuring antibody levels, lymphocyte immunophenotyping, and mutational analysis of the BTK gene. Patients invariably have low levels of IgA; most have low levels of IgG and IgM. B cells are absent by flow cytometry, distinguishing XLA from CVID. Carrier detection is available for women with a previously affected child or extended family members. Prenatal testing of male fetuses can also be done by chorionic villous sampling or by amniocentesis.

Treatment: Monthly IVIG, 400 to 600 mg/kg, is administered to maintain IgG trough levels over 500 mg/dL. Most male XLA patients are healthy while receiving IVIG-replacement therapy and experience normal growth and minimal sinopulmonary disease. Immunizations are unnecessary and are not indicated after replacement therapy is begun. Central nervous system symptoms require prompt diagnostic attention; enteroviral infections can be successfully treated with increased doses of IVIG, sometimes administered intrathecally. Lymphoreticular and gastrointestinal malignancy surveillance is required. Bacterial infections are treated with appropriate antimicrobial therapy.

Immunoglobulin Deficiency with Increased Levels of IgM

Immunoglobulin deficiency with normal or increased levels of IgM is a rare, inherited condition that is characterized by low levels of IgG, IgA, and IgE and normal or increased levels of IgM. Absence or defective expression of CD40 ligand, a surface molecule found on activated T cells, prevent isotype switching of B cells from IgM-secretory to IgA-, IgE-, and IgG-secreting cells. Fewer than 150 cases have been reported to date, and patients usually have been diagnosed in childhood. There is a high incidence of hepatic disease (e.g., sclerosing cholangitis, cirrhosis, and liver failure) associated with this disease, and there is also a high rate of malignancy. Treatment is with IVIG and pneumocystic prophylaxis. Some patients with nodular lymphoid hyperplasia, chronic diarrhea, and protein-losing enteropathy fail to respond to IVIG. Because of this and the risk of malignancy, bone marrow transplantation has been performed in approximately ten patients, with a current 50% success rate.

IgG Subclass Deficiency

Deficiencies of each of the four immunoglobulin subclasses (i.e., IgG1, IgG2, IgG3, and IgG4) occur in association with recurrent infections. The diagnosis is considered in patients with recurrent infections; normal total levels of IgG, IgA, and IgM; and decreased IgG subclass levels (lower than 2 SD below what is normal for age). IgG2 deficiency with or without IgA deficiency is the most common IgG subclass deficiency. Some subjects with IgG subclass deficiency are completely normal; therefore, the significance of isolated subclass deficiency is not clear. Two or more subclass deficiencies may coexist, such as IgG2 and IgG4 deficiency and IgG1 and IgG3 deficiency. Most patients with clinical illness have poor responses to diphtheria, tetanus toxoid, and pneumococcal immunizations.

Treatment: Prophylactic antimicrobial antibiotic therapy is appropriate for patients with IgG subclass deficiencies and recurrent infections. Amoxicillin or trimethoprim–sulfamethoxazole once or twice daily at half the treatment dose is usually beneficial. At this time, scientific evidence does not support the routine use of intravenous gammaglobulin–replacement therapy for isolated IgG subclass deficiency. There are reports of benefit in uncontrolled studies, but double-blind placebo-controlled studies are required. Consultation with a clinical immunologist–allergist is recommended.

Antibody Deficiency with Normal Immunoglobulins

Antibody deficiency with normal immunoglobulins is characterized by failure to produce protective levels of antibody in response to specific immunization, despite having normal or near-normal total serum immunoglobulin levels (6).

A relatively small published series of such patients suggests a role for immunoglobulin replacement therapy for such individuals.

Diagnosis: Patients with recurrent infections that are without a known cause who have normal serum levels of IgG, IgA, and IgM are considered for evaluation. Preimmunization pneumococcal antibody titers are obtained, and if protective titers are not present ($>$ 200 ng of antibody nitrogen per milliliter per serotype), patients should be immunized and their titers drawn at 4 weeks. Most adults develop protective antibody levels against serotypes 3, 7F, 9N, and 14. Prophylactic antibiotics for selected patients are indicated. A clinical immunologist–allergist should be consulted before immunoglobulin-replacement therapy is considered for selected patients who do not improve with antimicrobial therapy. IVIG is given for a finite period of time (e.g., 6 mo–1 y), with close monitoring to assess clinical benefits. Patients are then reassessed.

Combined Immunodeficiencies

The combined immunodeficiencies include the severe combined immunodeficiency diseases, major histocompatibility Class II deficiency, CD3+-activation deficiency, rare T-cell–activation deficiency, lymphokine deficiencies, Ommen syndrome, and DiGeorge syndrome. These diseases are almost exclusively diagnosed in infants and children; however, advances in treatment currently allow many such patients to survive into adult life. Medical management usually is provided in close consultation with the subspecialist.

Immunoglobulin-Replacement Preparations

The objectives of immunoglobulin replacement are to decrease the frequency and severity of infections and to improve the quality of life of patients with immunodeficiency diseases (7).

Intramuscular
Human serum immunoglobulin for intramuscular use comes as a 16% solution containing mostly IgG. Although intramuscular immunoglobulin-replacement therapy is effective and inexpensive, injections are painful and slowly absorbed, and high serum levels are not achieved.

Intravenous
Intravenous immunoglobulin preparations derived from human serum are comparable with respect to safety, antibody content, in vivo half-life, and clin-

---

Box 9.3 Adverse Reactions Associated with Immunoglobulin-Replacement Therapy

---

Vasodilatory and inflammatory
  Flushing, headache, nausea, vomiting, chest tightness, myalgias, hypertension
Anaphylactoid and anaphylaxis
Self-limited aseptic meningitis

---

ical efficacy. IVIG is available in 5%, 10%, and 12% solutions. IVIG has supplanted the intramuscular preparation, because higher dosages can be delivered with fewer side effects. Infusions are given according to a protocol, generally beginning at slow infusion rates (i.e., 0.5 mL/min) and then increasing incrementally to 150 to 300 cm^3/h. Vital signs are monitored regularly. Adverse reactions are listed in Box 9.3.

It is important that infusions be delivered by experienced personnel who are familiar with adverse-event management. Initial infusions usually are given in a hospital or office-based clinical facility. Patients who repeatedly tolerate infusions may receive infusions at home. Clinical assessments (e.g., infection frequency, antibiotic usage, and quality-of-life measures) should be performed on all patients. Trough IgG levels are obtained every 3 months and are required by third-party payers to document adequate replacement of IgG. Periodic liver function assessments are required. Transmission of viruses is of continual concern because IVIG is derived from 5000 to 10,000 blood-product donations. A small number of outbreaks of non-A, non-B (probably C) hepatitis have occurred and have been related to individual batches. There is no documented case of HIV having been transmitted by an immunoglobulin product. Because of manufacturers' efforts to apply new technologies in the preparation and testing of products, safety will probably improve with time. It is recommended that patients who receive IVIG replacement be followed by a specialist experienced in both the disease process and immunoglobulin therapy. Indications for IVIG in primary immunodeficiency diseases are listed in Box 9.4.

Phagocytic Disorders

Phagocytes, including neutrophils, monocytes and eosinophils, play an important role in the elimination of bacterial and fungal pathogens. Their function depends on coordinated actions of adherence, chemotaxis, granule function, and oxygen metabolism to allow effective phagocytosis of the organisms. X-linked and autosomal-recessive forms of the disease occur, and molecular

---

Box 9.4 Indications for Intravenous Immunoglobulin in Primary Immunodeficiency Disease

---

Primary antibody deficiency
  X-linked agammaglobulinemia
  Common variable hypogammaglobulinemia
  X-liked immunodeficiency with hyper-IgM
  Antibody deficiency with near normal immunoglobulins
  Combined immunodeficiency disease
Combined immunodeficiencies
  Primary Combined Cellular and Antibody Deficiency
  Severe Combined Immunodeficiency Disease
  Wiskott–Aldrich syndrome
  Ataxia telangiectasia
  X-linked lymphoproliferative syndrome
  Hyper-IgE syndrome

---

analyses have defined the genetic basis for the condition (8). The important task of the internist is to consider this diagnostic possibility in patients who present with an unusually severe manifestation of infection from common organisms (e.g., pyogenic liver abscess due to *Staphylococcus aureus*), recurrent infections with common bacterial pathogens, or infections with unusual pathogens (e.g., *Aspergillus fumigatus* or *Burkholderia cepecia*). Patients with recurrent viral infections or those with simple recurrent furunculosis do not require neutrophil functional evaluation.

Diagnosis

Most patients are diagnosed during childhood; however, some major defects present during adulthood. Familial history of severe infections or early deaths may be a helpful clue. Physical examination may show evidence of slow healing, poor scar formation, poor oral hygiene, poor dentition, gum recession, and gingivitis.

Treatment

The initial management problem is to classify and identify the functional defect by using specific laboratory tests that assess neutrophil function and that are carried out with the assistance of a clinical immunologist. Therapeutic modalities include the timely and aggressive use of antimicrobial therapy, chemoprophylaxis against further infection, genetic counseling, cytokine therapy (e.g., interferon-γ for the treatment of chronic granulomatous disease), and bone marrow transplantation.

Complement Deficiencies

Genetically determined complement deficiencies have been described for nearly all of the individual complement components, but they are rare (9). Clinical expressions include recurrent infections, rheumatic conditions, and angioedema. Patients with deficiencies of C3 (a major opsonin) experience recurrent infections of encapsulated bacteria, including *Streptococcus pneumoniae* and *H. influenzae*. Terminal components (C6789) are associated with gram-negative infections (e.g., *Neisseria meningitidis*), which are especially susceptible to the bactericidal activities of the complement system. The best screening test is the CH_{50}, which measures the ability of the patient's serum to lyse erythrocytes and which assesses the function of the components of the classical pathways. Complete absence of a component will result in a low CH_{50}.

Secondary Immunodeficiencies

Secondary immunodeficiencies are related to altered physiology that is associated with illness, age, nutrition, metabolic diseases, or adverse effects of medical therapies. AIDS secondary to HIV is the most prominent example, which is not within the scope of this review. The following discussion reviews aspects of secondary immunodeficiency important to the internist.

Aging

Infection ranks as the fourth leading cause of death for U.S. citizens over 65 years of age, and the eighth leading cause of death in those less than 65 years of age. Thymus gland involution is completed by approximately the fourth decade of life. Total lymphocyte counts and total IgG levels are maintained, but lymphocyte subpopulations and cytokine production are altered, which affects monocyte–macrophage function. Memory T cells outnumber naive cells; therefore, the repertoire of antigens to which the older person responds is limited. Decreased interleukin-2 production by T cells results in decreased proliferative capacity to antigens, including mycobacterial tuberculosis, varicella zoster, and influenza antigens. This is reflected by increased propensity for intracellular bacterial and viral diseases. Declining cell-mediated immunity to mycobacterium tuberculosis, and varicella-zoster is associated with increased reactivation frequency in elderly patients, clinical tuberculosis and shingles. Influenza immunization results in decreased antibody responses, and impaired cell-mediated immunity leads to delayed recovery from influenza infection (10).

Diagnosis and Treatment

No specific diagnostic tests to assess immunologic function are recommended routinely for the elderly, yet all patients over 65 years of age should be considered at increased risk for infection. Immunologic evaluations are indicated for those with recurrent, persistent infections or for those with an opportunistic processes. Tuberculin skin testing should be performed, especially in nursing home residents (who have a 3.5% skin-test conversion rate, even in the absence of known exposure), and appropriate chemoprophylaxis should be offered. Influenza immunizations are indicated for all elderly persons over 65 years of age who are not allergic to eggs.

Chemoprophylaxis with amantadine or ranitidine should be considered for those people who are immunized after community influenza A activity occurs in the autumn or early winter. Elderly patients with clinical influenza A are candidates for oral therapy with either drug. Such treatment reduces symptoms and fever by 1 to 2 days and provides more rapid overall functional recovery.

Case 9.2

A 64-year-old white man presented with an episode of pyelonephritis secondary to *Escherichia coli*. The patient reports fatigue over the previous 12 months and experienced two episodes of pneumonia that resolved with intravenous antibacterial therapy. His past medical history was unremarkable; social and family histories were deemed noncontributory. A review of systems revealed low back pain for 2 years.

His blood pressure, pulse rate, body temperature, and respiratory rate were all normal for his age. Results of examinations of the head, eyes, ears, and nose were normal; his throat was clear, and his neck was supple and without significant adenopathy. Results of chest, neurologic, cardiac, skin, abdominal, and rectal examinations were normal; there was no organomegaly present. Stool was negative.

Complete blood count revealed a white blood count of 15,000 (75% polymorphonuclear leukocytes; 6% bands; 12% lymphocytes; 3% monocytes). Hemoglobin was 9 g/dL. Electrolytes were within normal limits. Serum calcium levels were 10.7 mg/dL (8.8–10.5 mg/dL). Serum creatine levels were 1.7 mg/dL (0.8–1.4 mg/dL). Blood urea nitrogen levels were 27 mg/dL (5–25 mg/dL). The chest radiograph showed no abnormalities. In this case, evaluation of hypercalcemia, anemia, and renal insufficiency are considered in this context and favor systemic illness. Further diagnostic evaluation, including lumbosacral spine films and bone marrow examination, reveals lytic lesions. Serum protein electrophoresis demonstrates an M component. Bone marrow examination reveals plasmacytosis of greater than 10%. Serum im-

Case 9.2 (continued)

munoglobulins reveal IgG levels of 310 mg/dL (528–2190 mg/dL), IgA levels of 15 mg/dL (44–441 mg/dL), and IgM levels of 40 mg/dL (48–225 mg/dL). Tetanus, diphtheria, and pneumococcal titers are not protective following immunization.

This patient is a previously healthy adult with recurrent infections developing during the late middle years. Two episodes of pneumonia and pyelonephritis should alert the clinician to the possibility of primary immunodeficiency disease, such as CVID or secondary immunodeficiency associated with systemic illness (e.g., diabetes mellitus) and malignancy. This is a case of immunodeficiency secondary to multiple myeloma.

This patient will require therapeutic intervention directed by the hematologist–oncologist. Supportive care includes management of hypercalcemia, renal insufficiency, bone pain, and hyperviscosity. Pneumococcus is a dreaded pathogen in myeloma patients, and given the profound humoral immunodeficiency, one may consider intravenous gammaglobulin in selected cases. At this time, a consensus panel has recommended that intravenous gammaglobulin may have a role in patients with stable (plateau phase) disease and a high risk of recurrent infections (11).

Immunodeficiencies Secondary to Malignancies

Immunologic defects that are seen in patients with various cancers are listed in Box 9.5. Several lymphoid malignancies are associated with decreased antibody responses. Multiple myeloma results in decreased production and increased antibody metabolism; therefore, it is associated with infections of high-grade encapsulated bacterial pathogens, including *Streptococcus pneumoniae* and *H. influenzae*. Chronic lymphocytic leukemia in its advanced stages is often accompanied by hypogammaglobulinemia, and such patients suffer from sinopulmonary infections due to encapsulated bacteria. Patients with Hodgkin's disease demonstrate decreased delayed-type skin-test reactivity, but clinical infections usually are caused by encapsulated organisms (e.g., *S. pneumoniae, H. influenzae*), especially in those treated with radiotherapy, chemotherapy, and splenectomy.

The most common immunologic defects occurring in cancer patients are defects in the absolute number of neutrophils, which can occur in patients with leukemia and those treated with radiation or cytotoxic therapy. Neutropenia in these settings is associated with a high rate of bacteremia and rapidly progressive bacterial pneumonia. The normal lower limit for circulating neutrophils is 1500 cells/mm^3, and as counts fall below 500 cells/cm^3, there is an increased frequency of serious infections that correlates with the magnitude, rate, and duration of the neutrophil decline. Those with neutrophil counts below 100 are especially susceptible. Infections with *Candida* and *Aspergillus* species occur in addition to those bacterial pathogens.

Box 9.5 Immunologic Abnormalities That Occur in Patients with Malignancies

---

Decreased immunoglobulin synthesis
Decreased delayed-hypersensitivity skin tests
Decreased lymphocyte numbers
Decreased mitogen responses
Decreased production of cytokines
Decreased monocyte function

The pattern of infection may be modified by a number of factors, most notably indwelling catheters, endogenous flora, environmental exposures, use of prophylactic medications, concomitant humoral or cellular deficiencies, and other complicating conditions (e.g., hyperglycemia, uremia, and malnutrition).

Immunosuppressive Therapies

The common immunosuppressive therapies include irradiation, glucocorticosteroid administration, cytotoxic therapy, immunomodulating agents (e.g., cyclosporine and tacrolimus) and antilymphocyte antibodies. These therapies have broad immunosuppressive effects (8). Glucocorticosteroids are used for the treatment of the widest variety of illnesses and also produce the most significant adverse effects on immunologic function (Box 9.6).

The risk of infection secondary to treatment with glucocorticosteroids is related to dose and duration. Daily administration with doses of 20 to 40 mg over a 4- to 6-week period are sufficient. Primarily, infections are due to impaired phagocytic and cell-mediated immunity. A wide variety of organisms are pathogenic in such patients, including viruses, fungi, mycobacteria, staphylococci, gram-negative organisms, and *Nocardia* and *Listeria* species. The anti-inflammatory and immunosuppressive effects are less potent when glucocorticosteroids are given in alternate-day dosages, and serious infections do not occur often with such regimens.

Cyclosporine, tacrolimus, and azathioprine are potent immunosuppressive agents that predispose to opportunistic infections predominantly in transplantation recipients. Methotrexate given in low dosages (10–20 mg/wk) is used for the treatment of rheumatoid arthritis and in some patients with refractory asthma; it is associated with rare cases of *Pneumocystis carinii* and *Cryptococcus neoformans* infections. Cyclophosphamide (which is used for the treatment of malignancies, systemic lupus erythematous, Wegener's granulomatosis, and as conditioning therapy for bone marrow transplantation) suppresses cellular im-

> **Box 9.6 Immune-Related Adverse Effects of Patients with Gluco-corticosteroid Therapy**
>
> Impaired delayed hypersensitivity
> Decreased circulatory lymphocytes and monocytes
> Decreased monocyte responsiveness to chemoattraction
> Decreased neutrophil chemotaxis and microbial killing
> Decreased interferon production
> Impaired wound healing

munity and prevents antibody and autoantibody production. Bacterial and opportunistic infections occur in patients receiving cyclophosphamide, especially when it is given with daily glucocorticosteroids. Pulse-therapy dosage adjustments (to avoid extreme neutrophil nadirs) and alternate-day (rather than daily) administration of concomitant glucocorticosteroids reduce the incidence of infectious complications.

Immunodeficiencies Associated with Transplantation

Solid Organ Transplantation

Transplantation is an accepted treatment for kidney, liver, lung, and heart failure. Survival rates are improving such that living recipients with varying degrees of immune compromise now represent an increasing patient population. The types and severity of posttransplant infections vary with the organ transplanted, the level of immunosuppression, and the time course following transplantation. Postsurgical bacterial infections, line sepsis, and pneumonias predominate in the initial 4 weeks after transplantation. Opportunistic infections related to immunosuppression occur from 1 to 6 months after transplantation. Cytomegalovirus is a predominant pathogen. Clinical disease occurs most frequently in those treated with potent immunosuppressive agents, such as cyclophosphamide, cyclosporine, azathioprine, and anti–T-cell monoclonal antibodies. Clinical characteristics include prolonged fever, leukopenia, arthralgias, and hepatocellular enzyme injury. In the late posttransplant period, chronic viral infections and fungal infections occur, especially in transplant recipients who require high doses of immunosuppressive agents.

Bone Marrow Transplantation

Allogeneic bone marrow transplantation is widely used for treating a variety of hematologic malignancies, immunologic deficiencies, and aplastic anemia. Most recipients undergo pretransplant conditioning, which ablates marrow elements, rendering the patient profoundly immunodeficient and placing the patient at immediate risk for peritransplant infectious complications. Engraftment gradually occurs, with neutrophil counts rising above 1500 per cubic millimeter within 3 to 6 weeks in uncomplicated cases. Cellular and humoral reconstitution then gradually returns over 6 to 12 months. Graft-versus-host disease (GVHD) complicates transplantation in 40% to 80% of recipients, depending on the donor source (e.g., matched sibling, matched unrelated, cord blood), age of patient, number of T cells in the graft, and the GVHD prophylactic regimen. Patients with acute GVHD experience delayed immune reconstitution. The immune dysfunction is compounded by immunosuppressive therapy used to treat the GVHD. Chronic GVHD develops in 25% of transplanted patients, predominantly in those with moderate to severe acute GVHD. The nature of infectious complications following bone marrow transplantation is related to three phases of immune reconstitution. During the first few weeks after transplantation, bacterial infections are seen. Delay in reaching normal leukocyte counts predisposes the patient to invasive fungal infections, such as aspergillosis. Herpes simplex, cytomegalovirus, and *Pneumocystis carinii* pneumonia have been successfully prevented in most patients with the use of prophylactic antimicrobial regimens, although those recipients with GVHD remain at risk. Chronic GVHD results in chronic immunosuppression characterized by CD4+ lymphopenia and poor capacity for antibody production, resulting in persistent susceptibility to infection from high-grade encapsulated pathogens, such as *Streptococcus pneumoniae*. Varicella zoster also occurs in the late transplant period.

Immunodeficiencies Associated with Metabolic Diseases

A variety of metabolic and hereditary conditions are associated with the occurrence of recurrent infections. Specific immunologic defects accompany some of these (e.g., the cellular immunodeficiency that occurs in Down syndrome), and they should be identified. In other conditions, the infectious complications relate to pathologic changes not related to immune parameters (e.g., those occurring with diabetes mellitus), and diagnosis precludes the necessity for exhaustive immunologic evaluation. Box 9.7 lists the diseases associated with abnormalities of immune function and recurrent infections.

General Comments Regarding the Diagnosis of Immunodeficiencies

The diagnosis of immunodeficiencies is established with an accurate history, physical examination, and use of laboratory testing. Diagnostic tests should

Box 9.7 Metabolic and Hereditary Diseases

Diabetes mellitus	Iron deficiency
Sickle cell disease	Protein-losing enteropathy
Uremia	Congenital asplenia
Nephrotic syndrome	Down syndrome
Protein calorie malnutrition	

Table 9.1 Indications for Immunologic Evaluation*

One Episode	Two Episodes	Multiple Episodes
Osteomyelitis*	Sepsis	Sinusitis, bronchitis‡
Septic arthritis*	Pneumonia†	Pneumonia
Meningitis*		

* Immunologic work-up is not routinely necessary for isolated recurrent otitis media or recurrent genitourinary tract infections.
† Especially when pathogen is unusual
‡ In absence of atopy, smoking, and cystic fibrosis.

Table 9.2 Tests of Immunologic Function

	Humeral	Cellular	Phagocytic	Complement
Screening	IgG, IgA, IgM, IgE	Complete blood count Lymphocyte phenotyping Delayed-type hypersensitivity skin testing	Complete blood count Quantitative nitroblue tetrazoleum test	Total hemolytic complement (CH50)
Secondary	Antibody responses to diphtheria, tetanus, and pneumococcal immunizations Immunoglobulin subclass determination*	Lymphocyte proliferation in response to mitogens and antigens		Quantitation of complement components
Tertiary	Bacteriophage öX 174 neoantigen immunization response	Cytokine production	Phagocytosis and killing assay Chemotaxis	

* Significance not entirely clear at the time of this writing. Testing antibody responses to immunizations without obtaining subclasses is the preferable approach at this time.

be ordered in the most reliable and effective manner. Testing should be performed at an accredited laboratory that provides age-matched normal values. In general, consultation with a board-certified specialist in allergy and clinical immunology is recommended for testing beyond screening analyses. Patients who have one or both of the following should be considered for evaluation: 1) recurrent, persistent severe infections or infections with unusual pathogens; or 2) family history of immunodeficiency (Table 9.1).

Laboratory evaluation includes testing that ranges in complexity from screening tests to sophisticated analysis of specific immunologic functions. General screening should include complete blood count, erythrocyte sedimentation rate, tuberculin test and control, and consideration for chest and sinus radiographs. Screening immunologic tests for the four functional components are listed in Table 9.2.

REFERENCES

1. **World Health Organization Scientific Group.** Primary immunodeficiency diseases. Clin Exp Immunol. 1997;109(Suppl):1–28.

2. **Sicherer SH, Winkelstein JA.** Primary immunodeficiency diseases in adults. JAMA. 1998;279:58–61.

3. **Cunningham-Rundles C.** Disorder of the IgA system. In: Stiehm ER, ed. Immunologic Disorder in Infants and Children. 4th ed. Philadelphia: WB Saunders Co.; 1996:423–42.

4. **Rosen FS, Janeway CA.** The gamma globulins. Part III: The antibody deficiency syndromes. N Engl J Med. 1966;275:769–75.

5. **Vetrie D, Vorechovsky I, Sideras P, et al.** The gene involved in X-linked agammaglobulinemia is a member of the src family of protein-tyrosine kinases. Nature. 1993;361;226–33.

6. **French MA, Harrison G.** Systemic antibody deficiency in patients without serum immunoglobulin deficiency or with selective IgA deficiency. Clin Exp Immunol. 1984: 56;18–22.

7. **Polmar SH, Sorenson RO.** Immunoglobulin replacement therapy in primary immunodeficiency diseases. In: Rich RR, ed. Clinical Immunology Principles and Practice. St. Louis: Mosby; 1996:1865–75.

8. **Orkin SH.** Molecular genetics of chronic granulomatous disease. Ann Rev Immunol. 1989;7:277–307.

9. **Winkelstein JA, Sullivan KE, Colter HR.** Genetically determined deficiencies of complement. In: Metabolic Basis of Inherited Disease. New York City: McGraw-Hill; 1995:3912–41.

10. **Burns EA, Goodwin JS.** Immunodeficiency of aging. Drugs Aging. 1997:11:374–97.

11. **Ratko TA, Burnett DA, Foulke GE, et al.** Recommendations for off-label use of intravenously administered immunoglobulin preparations: University Hospital Consortium Expert Panel for Off-Label Use of Polyvalent Intravenously Administered Immunoglobulin Preparation. JAMA. 1995:273;1865–70.

SUGGESTED READINGS

Lawton AR, Hummell DS. Primary antibody deficiencies. In: Rich RR, ed. Clinical Immunology: Principles and Practice. v 1. St. Louis: Mosby; 1995:621–36.

Sicherer SH, Winkelstein JA. Primary immunodeficiency diseases in adults. JAMA. 1998;279:58–61.

World Health Organization Scientific Group. Primary immunodeficiency diseases. Clin Exp Immunol. 1997;109(Suppl):1–28.

Chapter 10

Allergen Immunotherapy

Roger W. Fox, MD

Richard F. Lockey, MD

Allergen immunotherapy—a series of allergen extract injections over a defined period of time—results in decreased sensitivity to inhaled or injected allergens, which can be measured both clinically and immunologically. Such therapy is used to treat allergic rhinitis (hay fever), allergic asthma, and stinging-insect hypersensitivity. During the first half of the century, efficacy of allergen immunotherapy was based primarily on clinical observations; however, over the past 40 years, scientific investigations of numerous allergens and of the complexities of the allergic reaction have unraveled the reasons for successful immunotherapy. This chapter reviews inhalant allergen immunotherapy used to treat allergic rhinitis and allergic asthma. Immunotherapy for stinging-insect hypersensitivity is covered in Chapter 6.

Overview of Practical Aspects

The overall clinical results of allergen immunotherapy in allergy practice is success. Reduction of symptoms and medication use is expected in the patient who has received the high-dose maintenance injections containing the relevant allergens for an appropriate period of 3 to 5 years. Generally, the allergist is the physician who provides the detailed prescription of the extract and the administration schedule. Careful selection of the patient and of the allergens for immunotherapy requires expertise and the knowledge about the pathophysiology of allergic diseases. The treating physician uses allergen immunotherapy in symptomatic patients who have failed environmental control measures and medications.

Allergens

Sources of aeroallergens include, but are not limited to, pollens, molds, and animal emanations (e.g., dander, saliva, urine, feces), and other animal parts derived from mammals, birds, insects, and house dust mites. Aeroallergens are able to induce a specific IgE-antibody response. This requires that the aeroallergen is sufficiently abundant in the ambient air to both sensitize and provoke allergic symptoms in a sensitized individual.

Ragweed-pollen–induced allergic rhinitis is an excellent model for aeroallergen-induced allergic diseases. First, the pollen is found in the air in sufficient quantities during the late summer and autumn pollinating season, and it is a potent sensitizer. Second, pollen induces symptoms in the sensitized patient during and immediately following the ragweed pollinating season. Third, ragweed-induced allergic rhinitis can be easily diagnosed both historically and by appropriate in vivo or in vitro testing for specific IgE to ragweed allergens.

The immediate effects of allergen exposure are readily observed in the ragweed-allergic patient during the ragweed pollinating season, as are the symptoms in the sensitized patient that are caused by an exposure to indoor allergens (e.g., those derived from dust mites, cats, and dogs). Such a temporal relationship is evidence of specific sensitivity; however, allergic symptoms also are caused by exposure to pollen and molds whose seasons overlap. Sometimes it is difficult, therefore, to ascertain which particular allergens are the most important as a cause of allergic disease. The physician must know which pollens, molds, and other aeroallergens are most important in the patient's geographic area. The American Academy of Allergy, Asthma, and Immunology has established a North American Pollen Network. Pollen and mold reports in various geographic areas are available by calling the National Allergy Bureau at 1-800-9-POLLEN or by writing to the American Academy of Allergy Asthma & Immunology, 611 East Wells Street, Milwaukee, WI 53202-3889.

Allergen Extracts

Licensing of allergenic products for clinical use in the United States is regulated by the Food and Drug Administration, Center for Biologics Evaluation and Research, Division of Allergenic Products and Parasitology. Many of the common extracts used in clinical allergy practice are available as standardized products or are pending standardization. This means that the allergen extract, as provided by commercial manufacturers, meets standards that ensure that the appropriate allergens are included in a given extract. Many allergen extracts, however, are not yet standardized, and it probably is not economically feasible or practical to standardize all of the extracts currently available for diagnosis and treatment.

Indications for Allergen Immunotherapy

Allergen avoidance, pharmacotherapy, and patient education form the basis for treating allergic rhinitis, conjunctivitis, and asthma. Allergen immunotherapy is indicated for patients with these diseases who have shown evidence of specific IgE antibodies to clinically relevant allergens. The indication for prescribing allergen immunotherapy depends on the degree to which symptoms can be reduced by allergen avoidance and by medication dose, type, and duration required to control symptoms. Immunotherapy, where appropriate, should be used with other forms of therapy. For stinging-insect–induced anaphylaxis, specific immunotherapy with Hymenoptera venom extract is the treatment of choice (*see* Chapter 6).

Controlled studies demonstrate that allergen immunotherapy is effective treatment for patients with respiratory allergies (Table 10.1). Immunotherapy is specific for the allergen administered, and the content of the treatment extract is based on the patient's history and allergy test results. In general, the very young and elderly patients are not candidates for immunotherapy. The very young patient with respiratory allergic diseases usually responds favorably to environmental control and pharmacotherapy; an uncooperative child is not the ideal candidate for allergen injections. The elderly patient rarely requires immunotherapy for the management of rhinitis, asthma, or both, because inhalant allergens usually are not the cause of respiratory symptoms in this age group. The optimal duration of immunotherapy to achieve the best therapeutic response remains un-

Table 10.1 Summary of Controlled Trials of Immunotherapy

	Allergic Rhinitis	Asthma
Grass	++	+
Weed	++	++
Tree	++	+
Molds	+	+/–
Mites	++	+
Cat dander	++	++
Dog dander	+	+

– = no effect; + = positive effect; ++ = strong positive effect

known; however, several studies indicate that 3 to 5 years of immunotherapy for patients who have had a good therapeutic response is adequate (1).

Immunologic Changes
Induced by Allergen Immunotherapy

The commonly recognized immunologic changes that occur secondary to successful allergen immunotherapy (Box 10.1) include 1) a rise in serum IgG-"blocking" antibody; 2) a blunting of the usual seasonal rise of IgE, followed by a slow decline of IgE over the course of immunotherapy; 3) an increase in IgG- and IgA-blocking antibodies in the respiratory mucosal secretions; 4) a reduction in basophil reactivity and sensitivity to specific allergens; and 5) reduced lymphocyte responsiveness (proliferation and cytokine production) to specific allergens (1).

The hallmark of asthma and allergic rhinitis is allergic inflammation of the mucosa and submucosa, predominantly caused by eosinophils. Th2 lymphocytes amplify and prolong allergic inflammation and late-phase reactions. Th1 cytokines (i.e., IFN-γ and IL-2) inhibit production of Th2 cytokines. Success-

---

Box 10.1 Proposed Sequence of Events for Successful Immunotherapy

Step 1: Suppression of the inflammatory-cell response to allergen prior to measurable immunologic changes
  Reduced cellular activation and mediator release
  Rapid changes in target organ mast cells, basophils, and eosinophils
Step 2: Production of IgG blocking antibodies
  IgG1 subclass antibodies early in the course
  IgG4 subclass antibodies predominate later in the course
Step 3: Suppression of IgE response to seasonal and other allergens
  Blunting of seasonal rise of IgE
  Gradual decline of specific allergen IgE
Step 4: Alteration of the controlling T-cell lymphocytes
  Down-regulation of Th2 lymphocyte cytokine profile
  Down-regulation of IgE antibody production and eosinophil activation
Step 5: Reduction of target organ hypersensitivity and mast cell and basophil cellular sensitivity
  Reduced cellular hypersensitivity
  Reduced biologic responses

ful immunotherapy might be associated with a shift in IL-4/IFN-γ production (from IL-4 to IFN-γ) either as a consequence of down-regulation of Th2 response or an increase in Th1 response. The exact mechanism involved in this favorable down-regulation of allergic inflammation is unknown (2).

Not all immunologic changes associated with effective immunotherapy occur in all subjects, although there is a general correlation between clinical improvement and the alteration of various immunologic parameters. This reduction in biologic sensitivity to specific allergens has been demonstrated in allergen immunotherapy trials to such allergens as 1) ragweed, mixed grasses, birch, and mountain-cedar–pollen extracts; 2) the molds *Alternaria* and *Cladosporium*; 3) cat dander; and 4) house dust mites. Successful allergen immunotherapy ameliorates, but usually does not completely eliminate, the respiratory symptoms of allergic rhinitis and allergic asthma.

Clinical Trials and Scientific Studies

Allergic Rhinitis: Overview

Many randomized, double-blind, controlled trials for allergic rhinitis due to airborne pollens, animal allergens, and house dust mite aeroallergens demonstrate efficacy of allergen immunotherapy based on subjective symptom scores and medication diaries. Favorable immunologic changes include decreased basophil histamine release, reduced skin-test allergen reactivity, and increased allergen-specific IgG-blocking antibody.

Pollens
Nasal challenge studies enable investigators to measure the allergic response in the upper airway following allergen immunotherapy. Such research demonstrates that there is a dose response to ragweed allergen immunotherapy, i.e., an optimal dose above which no additional improvement occurs. The first of these studies involved 12 ragweed-sensitive subjects who received immunotherapy with the principal ragweed-pollen allergen Antigen E (AgE; now known as *Amb a 1*). Injections were given for 3 to 5 years, and results were compared with those from 27 untreated control subjects. Nasal provocation studies of treated subjects revealed that AgE immunotherapy decreased the clinical response to ragweed and decreased the allergic inflammatory mediator responses (e.g., histamine, prostaglandin D2, TAME-esterase, and kinins) to an intranasal ragweed challenge. In a later study, 26 previously non-immunized ragweed-sensitive subjects were randomized to three different dosage regimens (low to high doses; 0.6–25.0 μg AgE injection), and their responses to ragweed nasal challenges were compared. The low-dose im-

munotherapy regimen provided no protective effect, whereas the moderate- and high-dose regimens caused significantly reduced mediator release from the nasal mucosa following ragweed nasal challenge. Symptom scores, which were recorded by the moderate- and high-dose treated subjects over three ragweed seasons, also improved significantly and correlated with the decreased release of inflammatory mediators. There was no significant difference in the degree of clinical improvement between the moderate- and high-dose groups. An example of a typical immunotherapy schedule needed to achieve an optimal immunotherapy dose is found in Table 10.2.

Nasal challenges also confirm that such therapy attenuates both the immediate and late-phase allergic responses by decreasing mucosal membrane cellular influx and mediator production. Ragweed immunotherapy for 3 to 5 years is required to achieve clinical remission. Both mixed- and single-

Table 10.2 Illustrative Dose Schedule for Short Ragweed-Allergen Immunotherapy

Dose Number	Vial	Dilution of 1:10 Weight: Volume Concentration*	Dose (mL)	Ragweed Amb a I (µg)
1	D	1:100,000	0.05	
2	D	1:100,000	0.10	
3	D	1:100,000	0.20	
4	D	1:100,000	0.30	
5	D	1:100,000	0.40	
6	C	1:10,000	0.05	
7	C	1:10,000	0.10	
8	C	1:10,000	0.20	
9	C	1:10,000	0.30	
10	C	1:10,000	0.40	
11	B	1:1000	0.05	
12	B	1:1000	0.10	
13	B	1:1000	0.20	
14	B	1:1000	0.30	
15	B	1:1000	0.40	
16	A	1:100	0.05	
17	A	1:100	0.10	Desirable
18	A	1:100	0.20	dose range
19	A	1:100	0.30	of 3–12 µg
20	A	1:100	0.40	

*A ratio of 1:10 weight:volume means that 1 g of pure pollen is diluted in 10 mL of diluent; 1:10 weight:volume extract of standardized ragweed extract contains 400 µg/m of Amb a I (Antigen E). Maintenance dose of immunotherapy is administered on a weekly to monthly schedule but can be altered on an individual basis. The table shows a weekly injection schedule (weeks 1–20). More rapid build-up can be accomplished by giving the injections twice weekly or by using a "rush" immunotherapy protocol, which achieves maintenance doses in days rather than weeks.

grass–pollen immunotherapy studies for hay fever result in significantly decreased symptom-medication scores during the grass-pollen season and responses to grass skin testing and nasal challenge testing. Increases in grass-specific IgG-blocking antibodies occur in subjects successfully treated with mixed grass immunotherapy. The size of the reaction to both the immediate and late-phase skin tests to timothy-grass extract was diminished in a timothy-allergen immunotherapy study.

Immunotherapy with mountain-cedar–pollen extract reduces the late-phase skin-test reaction to mountain-cedar–pollen extract and, during the cedar-pollen season, decreases symptom-medication scores, increases serum levels of the specific IgG, and decreases the seasonal rise in specific IgE. Similar clinical and immunologic results were obtained in immunotherapy trials with birch-pollen extract. In addition, birch-pollen nasal provocation studies showed inhibition of allergic symptoms and reduced chemotactic activities for eosinophils and neutrophils in nasal secretions after allergen immunotherapy.

Mites, Molds, and Animal Danders

Immunotherapy with house dust mite allergen results in significantly decreased nasal symptom scores, responses to nasal allergen challenge, and the size of the skin-test reaction. The same changes in specific serum levels of IgG and IgE as observed with pollen studies were found. *Alternaria* mold immunotherapy produces similar decreases in nasal-symptom–medication scores, allergen-provocative challenges in the skin and nose, and increased serum IgG levels. Cat allergen immunotherapy results in reduced nasal symptom scores of subjects exposed to a cat in a study room.

Allergic Asthma: Overview

More than 50 controlled immunotherapy trials have been performed with a variety of allergens for seasonal, perennial, and animal-induced asthma (3,4). Extracts of rye grass, mixed grasses, ragweed, birch, mountain cedar, *Alternaria*, *Cladosporium*, house dust mite, cat, dog, and cockroach have been used in these trials. Collective analysis of these studies provides important insight, but comparisons among studies are difficult because of varied study designs. Of these studies, 42 demonstrated significant clinical improvement in treated subjects. Twenty-three showed a significant increase in the bronchoprovocation threshold to the allergen extract used for immunotherapy. Of the trials in which immunologic parameters were monitored, 16 demonstrated an increase in allergen-specific IgG-blocking antibody, and one showed a decline in specific IgE. Nine reported decreased skin-test reactivity to the allergen used for immunotherapy, and two demonstrated reduced in vitro basophil histamine release following allergen challenge. An overall analysis of controlled studies

in the treatment of asthma with allergen immunotherapy indicates clinical efficacy in selected allergic asthmatics.

A meta-analysis of most of the controlled trials of allergen immunotherapy
for asthma that were published in the *American Journal of Respiratory and Critical
Care Medicine* in 1995 (5) indicates that allergen immunotherapy is effective in
the treatment of allergic asthma, provided that the clinically relevant and unavoidable allergen can be identified. The arguments favoring immunotherapy
are especially strong in the case of younger patients who require year-round
medical management. If allergen immunotherapy is elected, it should be administered in sufficiently high doses to maximize the benefits. With these optimal doses, there is the expectation of a reduction in medication requirements
and symptom scores in the majority of treated patients.

The National Heart, Lung, and Blood Institute (NHLBI) in 1997 spon-
sored an expert panel to establish guidelines for the diagnosis and management of asthma. This national asthma education and prevention program
states that 75% to 85% of patients are allergic and that immunotherapy should
be considered in such patients when avoidance of allergens and treatment
with appropriate medications does not control the disease.

Pollens

Allergic asthmatic subjects often experience increased bronchial hyperactivity
during a specific pollen season. The effect of birch-pollen immunotherapy on
bronchial reactivity, as measured by methacholine provocation, was investigated in subjects with birch-pollen asthma induced during the birch-pollen
season. Untreated subjects had increased bronchial hyperreactivity to methacholine, whereas those on birch-pollen immunotherapy did not. In addition,
eosinophil cationic protein—an inflammatory mediator derived from
eosinophils in the bronchoalveolar lavage fluid—was decreased in subjects receiving birch-pollen immunotherapy. Other studies using immunotherapies of
mixed grasses, cedar, birch, mugwort, and ragweed pollens demonstrate reduced bronchial responses to methacholine or histamine.

The benefits of immunotherapy are specific for the allergen(s) used in treatment. Some studies have shown that single-pollen immunotherapy (e.g., allergen derived from one grass species) may provide incomplete relief of
asthmatic symptoms because of multiple-grass sensitivity or because other
sensitivities (e.g., to molds) exist. Similarly, highly purified, standardized ragweed-allergen extract containing only a single-protein allergen (e.g., ragweed
AgE or *Amb a 1*) may provide incomplete relief of symptoms in patients with
ragweed-sensitive asthma, because they are sensitized to several ragweed proteins and not just AgE.

The IgE immune response differs between asthmatic patients who are polysensitized and those who are monosensitized. Patients sensitized to a single

allergen have significantly lower total serum IgE levels than those allergic to multiple allergens. The lymphocytes from the polysensitized subject, when challenged with allergen, release significantly more interleukin (IL) 4 and CD23 in vitro than those from the monosensitized subject, although the lymphocyte interferon-γ (IFN-γ) in vitro production is the same in both groups.

One double-blind placebo-controlled study performed during the pollen season compared the efficacy of immunotherapy in monosensitized (orchard-grass pollen) and polysensitized (multiple pollens, including orchard grass) asthmatic subjects (4). Subjects who were allergic to grass-pollen extract were treated with an optimal maintenance dose of a standardized orchard-grass–pollen extract, whereas those allergic to multiple pollen species, including grass, received the same biologically equivalent dose of all standardized allergens to which they were sensitized. The results indicated that subjects with orchard-grass–pollen allergy—but not polysensitized subjects—were significantly protected during the respective pollen season. If the results of this single study are verified, then sustained and higher doses of standardized extract may be required to demonstrate efficacy in polysensitized allergic patients.

A 5-year study of the role of immunotherapy in ragweed-induced asthma was published in 1993 (6). Clinical parameters (e.g., symptom-diary scores, medication use, measurements of peak expiratory flow rate, physician evaluations) and other end points (e.g., skin test sensitivity, serologic parameters, bronchial sensitivity to ragweed and methacholine) were monitored. A standardized maintenance dose of ragweed extract containing *Amb a 1* (10 µg per injection) was used to immunize ragweed-sensitive subjects. Both clinical and objective parameters improved, demonstrating that the use of an appropriate therapeutic dose is necessary to achieve a good clinical response.

In 1996, Creticos and coworkers (7) examined the efficacy of allergen immunotherapy for asthma exacerbated by seasonal ragweed exposure. Sixty-four patients completed 1 year of the study treatment, and 53 patients completed 2 years. These patients were not exclusively ragweed sensitive. Compared with the placebo group, the immunotherapy group had increased IgG antibodies to ragweed and reduced hay fever symptoms, skin-test sensitivity to ragweed, and sensitivity to bronchial challenges. The seasonal increase in IgE antibodies to ragweed allergen was abolished in the immunotherapy group after 2 years. The patients received doses of 4 µg of *Amb a 1* per injection during the 1st year and 10 µg per injection the 2nd year.

Although positive effects were observed in the immunotherapy asthma group, the clinical effects were limited. Both immunotherapy and placebo groups had some improvement in asthma symptoms during the study.

In 1997, Adkinson and coworkers (8) performed a controlled trial of immunotherapy for asthma in allergic children. A placebo-controlled trial of multiple-allergen immunotherapy in 121 allergic children with moderate to severe perennial asthma was conducted over 2 years. The median medication-score decline was not significantly different between the immunotherapy and placebo groups. The numbers of days on oral corticosteroids were similar in the two groups, and there was no difference between the groups as to the use of medical care, symptoms, or peak flow rates. Partial or complete remission of asthma occurred in 31% of the immunotherapy group and in 28% of the placebo group. The median PC_{20} for methacholine (which is the amount of methacholine needed to cause a decrease of $\geq 20\%$ in the forced expiratory volume in 1 s [FEV_1]) increased significantly in both groups, but there was no difference between the two study groups. Optimal doses of immunotherapy, ranging from 4.3 to 26.0 μg per injection, resulted in a mean 8.8-fold increase in the levels of allergen-specific IgG to *Dermatophagoides pteronyssinus*, *D. farinae*, short ragweed, oak, and grass. A 61% mean reduction in wheal diameters by prick skin testing to each respective allergen was observed. The groups that most benefited from immunotherapy were children with milder disease (no inhaled corticosteroids) and younger children (< 8.5 y of age) with a shorter duration of disease. Overall, the data indicated no discernible benefit in allergic children with perennial asthma from immunotherapy who were already receiving appropriate and optimal medical treatment from asthma experts.

Mites

Various studies of immunotherapy with extracts of standardized aqueous *D. pteronyssinus*, *D. farinae*, or both demonstrated significant benefit. A study by Bousquet and Michel (4) revealed that among subjects allergic only to *D. farinae*, children showed a significantly greater improvement than did adults. As expected, patients with severe, chronic asthma ($FEV_1 \leq 70\%$ of predicted), other perennial allergen sensitivities, aspirin intolerance, or chronic sinusitis achieved the least benefit from immunotherapy.

Another study by Bousquet and Michel (9) analyzed immunotherapy to *D. pteronyssinus* in 74 mite-allergic asthma patients. It demonstrated a significantly increased dose-dependent tolerance to the standardized *D. pteronyssinus* allergen, *Der p* I, on bronchial allergen challenge in each of the immunized groups versus no change in the control group. A significant reduction in histamine bronchoprovocation hyper-responsiveness also was observed, with the greatest reduction occurring in the highest dose group. The rate of systemic reactions was lowest in the low-dose group and highest in the high-dose group, and because the 7- and 21-μg-per-injection schedules were equally effective, the 7-μg-per-injection dose was recommended as the appropriate target dose.

Danders

Several controlled studies found that cat and dog immunotherapy effectively increases the threshold dose of cat- or dog-dander extract needed to induce a positive bronchial challenge in subjects with cat- or dog-specific allergic asthma. Such therapy also results in a reduction of symptoms after dander exposure in a challenge room. Many subjects are given cat or dog immunotherapy at their own request in an effort to better tolerate the presence of a pet in their home; however, confirmation of clinical efficacy under such circumstances is needed, and elimination of the animal from the environment in which the subject lives is the preferable mode of therapy (10).

Molds

Molds that trigger asthma are numerous, diverse, and contain multiple allergens. Mold extracts available for use in the United States are not standardized. Controlled immunotherapy trials with standardized extracts of *Alternaria* and *Cladosporium* demonstrate efficacy in the treatment of asthma. One such trial of 1-year treatment with *Alternaria* resulted in ablation or a reduced late-phase response upon *Alternaria*-allergen challenge in 8 of 10 subjects. Increased concentrations of allergen and methacholine also were required to induce bronchial constriction. *Cladosporium herbarium*–extract immunotherapy produced significant decreases in symptom-medication scores and in response to bronchial challenge tests. Many of the same in vitro changes were observed in this study.

Reasons for Lack of Benefit from Immunotherapy

The reasons for lack of benefit from allergen immunotherapy include 1) the inappropriate treatment with such therapy of non–IgE-mediated disease (e.g., chronic nonallergic rhinitis, vasomotor rhinitis) (6); 2) use of low-potency allergen extracts; 3) inadequately administered doses of allergen; 4) ineffective environmental control, resulting in continued excessive exposure (e.g., to cat or dog dander); 5) coexistent medical problems (e.g., sinusitis and nasal polyps) accounting for most symptoms; and 6) allergen extract lacking important constituents due to undiagnosed or unrecognized sensitivities.

Duration of Immunotherapy

An advantage of allergen immunotherapy versus pharmacotherapy is that the former down-regulates the abnormal immunologic responses that cause allergic respiratory diseases. Clinical impressions and observations suggest that treatment can be stopped after 3 to 5 years of successful therapy. Naclerio and coworkers (11) demonstrated continued suppression of allergic rhinitis symptoms after discontinuation of ragweed immunotherapy. Immunologic parameters and nasal lavage mediators remained essentially unchanged 1 year after cessation of therapy in most subjects. The mechanism responsible for continued efficacy is unknown. Patients who relapse after discontinuation of immunotherapy can resume their previous successful immunotherapy regimen.

Adverse Reactions

Local Reactions

Patients receiving allergen immunotherapy often experience reactions at the site of the injection (e.g., erythema and edema), which cause some discomfort to the patient. No adjustment in extract dose is necessary for reactions less than 4 mm in size. Large local reactions ($>$ 4 cm in diameter) occur less frequently but may cause more discomfort and persist for 24 hours or longer. There is a concern that subsequent increases in the dose of the extract following a large local reaction may result in a systemic reaction; however, there is little evidence that such local reactions, whatever their size, place the subject at increased risk for a systemic reaction. This local discomfort can be controlled with cold compresses and oral antihistamines. When such reactions occur, the subsequent allergen-immunotherapy dose usually is reduced to the previously tolerated dose and subsequently increased. If large local reactions persist, divide the dose into two separate doses given at different sites.

Systemic Reactions

Systemic reactions occur rarely and may be mild (e.g., manifested as generalized pruritus, urticaria, or symptoms of allergic rhinitis and conjunctivitis) or life-threatening, with upper and lower airway obstruction, anaphylactic shock, or both. Fatalities are rare but do occur. A retrospective questionnaire survey of allergy specialists in the United States for the period 1945 to 1983 reported 46 fatalities either from skin testing or immunotherapy (12). The data given for 30 of these fatalities allowed for further evaluation: Six were caused by skin testing and 24 by immunotherapy. A later extension of this study included reports of an additional 17 deaths between 1985 and 1989. Further reporting through 1995 has disclosed another 27 fatalities related to immunotherapy.

In 1997, the Mayo Clinic reported on their more than 10 years of experience with immunotherapy. The incidence of reactions was low (0.137%); most were mild and responded to immediate medical intervention, and there were no fatalities. The estimated fatality rate from allergen immunotherapy in the United States was approximately one for every two million injections for the period between 1985 and 1989. Risk factors cited in this group were active asthma and having been increased to a higher-dose immunotherapy. Bousquet's observations in his asthma immunotherapy trials (4,9) were that mite-sensitive individuals had more immunotherapy-related asthma reactions than those who were pollen sensitive. He commented that fewer reactions occurred on maintenance than during the build-up phase. Excluding the severe or unstable asthmatic from receiving the immunotherapy injections significantly reduced the rate of systemic reactions.

Precautions

No allergen extract should be considered completely safe for an allergic patient, and immunotherapy should be carried out only by trained personnel who know how to administer immunotherapy injections, adjust doses, and manage adverse reactions in a setting in which appropriate equipment for such management is immediately available.

Patients at higher risk for a severe life-threatening systemic reaction are listed in Box 10.2. Pregnant patients who are already receiving immunotherapy may be maintained at their current or reduced dose during pregnancy. Initiating immunotherapy during pregnancy is not advisable unless a life-threatening situation exists, such as a patient with Hymenoptera hypersensitivity who cannot avoid the possibility of being re-stung. Relative contraindications for immunotherapy include noncompliance, severe psychiatric disorders, and autoimmune or immunodeficiency diseases.

Box 10.2 Patients at Higher Risk for Severe Life-Threatening Systemic Reactions

---

Patients with unstable or symptomatic asthma

Patients with significant seasonal exacerbation of their allergic symptoms, particularly asthma

Patients with a high degree of hypersensitivity (by skin testing or specific IgE measurements)

Patients on accelerated schedules of immunotherapy, particularly during the initial build-up period

Patients on high-dose maintenance regimens (in highly sensitive allergic patients)

Patients concomitantly using β-blockers, which makes treatment of anaphylaxis with epinephrine more difficult; β-blockers should be discontinued before initiating immunotherapy, when possible

Patients receiving injections from new vials

The risk of systemic allergic reactions and fatal reactions should be reduced and, hopefully, eliminated by 1) avoiding errors in dosing; 2) using preventive protocols to minimize risk, such as measuring peak flow rates in patients with unstable asthma; 3) reducing doses when giving injections from new vials; 4) reducing doses when giving injections during seasonal exacerbations; and 5) using standardized allergen extracts.

Any physician who administers immunotherapy, regardless of specialty, should be present when the injections are given. The patient should be required to stay in the office 20 minutes following the injection. A longer wait may be indicated for high-risk patients. In the event of any adverse reactions or uncertainty about the dose, the allergist should be consulted before administration of another dose of allergen extract.

Treatment of Allergic Reactions: Medications and Equipment

Physicians prescribing or administering immunotherapy must be aware of the potential risks and institute appropriate office procedures to minimize them (13). The prompt recognition of signs and symptoms of a systemic reaction and the immediate use of epinephrine to treat such a reaction are the mainstays of therapy. The following equipment, medications, and reagents should be available: 1) stethoscope and sphygmomanometer; 2) tourniquets, syringes, hypodermic needles, and large-bore (14-gauge) needles; 3) aqueous epinephrine hydrochloride (1:1000 weight:volume); 4) equipment to administer oxygen; 5) equipment to administer intravenous fluids; 6) oral airway; 7) antihistamines; 8) corticosteroids; and 9) injectable vasopressor.

Current and Future Trends in Immunotherapy

Advances in basic immunology should lead to new, safer, and more effective methods to alter the human immune response. Many of the important allergens have been cloned, key epitopes have been identified, and modified allergens are being investigated. Recombinant DNA technology allows for the large-scale production of highly purified and defined allergens for diagnostic and therapeutics purposes. New forms of immunotherapy to treat allergic diseases include recombinant DNA technology and synthetic allergen-derived peptides. A key mechanism for successful conventional immunotherapy may be to alter T-cell function by diminishing production of Th2 cytokines, by inducing "immune deviation" from a Th2 cytokine pattern to a Th1 pattern, or both. One strategy includes the use of safe allergen derivatives that stimulate the favorable lymphocyte response, without the potential of causing anaphylaxis. Isoforms of major allergens have been identified that show no or very low IgE-binding capacity but contain T-cell–stimulating sequences. This type of peptide immunotherapy may represent an effective low-risk alternative to traditional immunotherapy. In peptide immunotherapy, the allergen is split into smaller pieces of 15 to 27 amino acids. By preserving only fragments of the allergen molecule that induces an immunologic response, triggering mast cell perturbation is avoided.

Another approach is to create nonanaphylactic IgE-binding haptens that might be used to saturate the effector cells, such as the mast cell, locally to prevent subsequent activation by exposure to the complete allergen. Perhaps the generation of IgG-blocking antibodies directed against the same IgE epitopes may accomplish desensitization. Intramuscular injection of plasmid DNA, which contains DNA encoding for a specific allergen, is an alternative to the injection of the antigen itself. Transfection of host cells will elicit humoral and cytoxic lymphocyte-mediated responses.

Research endeavors suggest that specific IgG antibodies block IgE binding and inhibit histamine release in allergic patients. IgG-blocking antibodies may be used to reduce IgE-mediated allergic reactions; therefore, recombinant allergen-specific F(ab′)2 fragments (those that bind to mast cell receptors) may be useful for passive blocking therapy of IgE-mediated allergic reactions. Recombinant F(ab′)2 fragments can be produced in bacterial expression systems. Other strategies include developing humanized anti-IgE monoclonal antibodies and induction of autoantibodies against the IgE-receptor binding site.

Chemically modified allergens have been tested in allergic subjects. Results demonstrate that glutaraldehyde- or polyethylene glycol–modified allergen extracts are effective and that fewer injections are necessary with these modified extracts compared with conventional aqueous extracts. Chemically modified allergens for immunotherapy have not been licensed by the Food and Drug Administration.

Given the extensive evidence that T cells play an important role in allergic disease, it seems logical to develop novel targets of immunotherapy that directly affect the T cell. Such innovative approaches are not yet approved for use in clinical practice.

REFERENCES

1. **Ohman JL Jr.** Clinical and immunologic responses to immunotherapy. In: Lockey RF, Bukantz SC, eds. Allergen Immunotherapy. New York: Marcel Dekker, Inc.; 1991:209–32.
2. **Bush RK, Ritter MW.** Allergen immunotherapy for the allergic patient. Immunol Allergy Clin North Am. 1992;12:107–24.

3. **Fox RW, Lockey RF.** Role of Immunotherapy in Asthma. In: Gershwin ME, Halpern GM, eds. Bronchial Asthma: Principles of Diagnosis and Treatment. 3rd ed. Totowa, NJ: Humana Press; 1994:365–98.

4. **Bousquet J, Michel FB.** Specific immunotherapy in asthma: is it effective? J Allergy Clin Immunol. 1994;94:1–11.

5. **Abramson MJ, Puy RM, Weiner JM.** Is allergen immunotherapy effective in asthma? A meta-analysis of randomized controlled trials. Am J Respir Crit Care Med. 1995;151:969–74.

6. **Creticos PS, Reed CE, Norman PS.** The NIAID cooperative study of the role of immunotherapy in seasonal ragweed-induced adult asthma. J Allergy Clin Immunol. 1993;91:226.

7. **Creticos PS, Reed CE, Norman PS, et al.** Ragweed immunotherapy in adult asthma. N Engl J Med. 1996;334:501–6.

8. **Adkinson NK, Eggleston PA, Eney D, et al.** A controlled trial of immunotherapy for asthma in allergic children. N Engl J Med. 1997;336:32–31.

9. **Bousquet J, Michel FB.** Specific immunotherapy in allergic rhinitis and asthma. In: Busse WW, Holgate ST, eds. Rhinitis and Asthma. Boston: Blackwell Scientific Publications; 1994:1309–24.

10. **Van Metre TE, Adkinson NF.** Immunotherapy for aeroallergen disease. In: Middleton E, Reed CE, Ellis EF, et al., eds. Allergy Principles and Practices. 4th ed. Baltimore, MD: Mosby; 1997:1489–1506.

11. **Naclerio RM, Proud D, Moylan B, et al.** Clinical aspects of allergic disease: a double-blind study of the discontinuation of ragweed immunotherapy. J Allergy Clin Immunol. 1997;100:293–300.

12. **Lockey RF, Benedict LM, Turkeltaub PC, Bukantz SC.** Fatalities from immunotherapy and skin testing. J Allergy Clinic Immunol. 1987;79:660–7.

13. **Joint Task Force on Practice Parameters.** Practice parameters for allergen immunotherapy. J Allergy Clin Immunol. 1996;98:1001–11.

SUGGESTED READINGS

Bosquet J, Hejjaoui A, Dhivert H, et al. Immunotherapy with the standardized *Dermatophagoides pteronyssinus* extract. Part III: Syestemic reactions during the rush protocol in patients suffering from asthma. J Allergy Clin Immunol. 1989;83:797–802.

Bosquet J, Lockey RF, Malling HJ (eds). World Health Organization positionn paper. Allergen immunotherapy: therapeutic vaccines for allergic diseases. Eur J Allergy Clin Immunol. 1998;44:1–42.

Lockey RF, Bukantz SC (eds). Allergens and allergen immunotherapy. In Clinical Allergy and Immunology. 2nd ed. New York: Marcel Dekker; 1999.

Platts-Mills TAE, Chapman MD. Allergen standardization [Editorial]. J Allergy Clin Immunol. 1991;3:621–4.

Index